Down on James Street

By Nicole McCandless

Illustrations by Byron Gramby

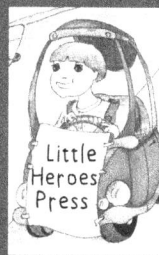

Down on James Street

Copyright © 2021 by Nicole McCandless.

No part of this book may be reproduced or transmitted in any form or by an electronic or mechanical means, including photocopying, recording or by any information storage and retrieval system, without the express written permission of the publisher, except where permitted by law.

Published by Hard Ball Press.

Information available at: www.hardballpress.com

ISBN 978-1-7344938-6-3

Story by Nicole McCandless

Illustrations by Byron Gramby

Cover Photo by Byron Gramby

Exterior & Interior design by Josephine O'Neil

Library of congress Cataloging-in-publication data
1. Children – fiction. 2. Pittsburgh – fiction. 3. Civil rights –fiction. 4. Black Lives Matter - fiction

*This book is dedicated to all the kids
who are still dancing and still fighting for justice.*

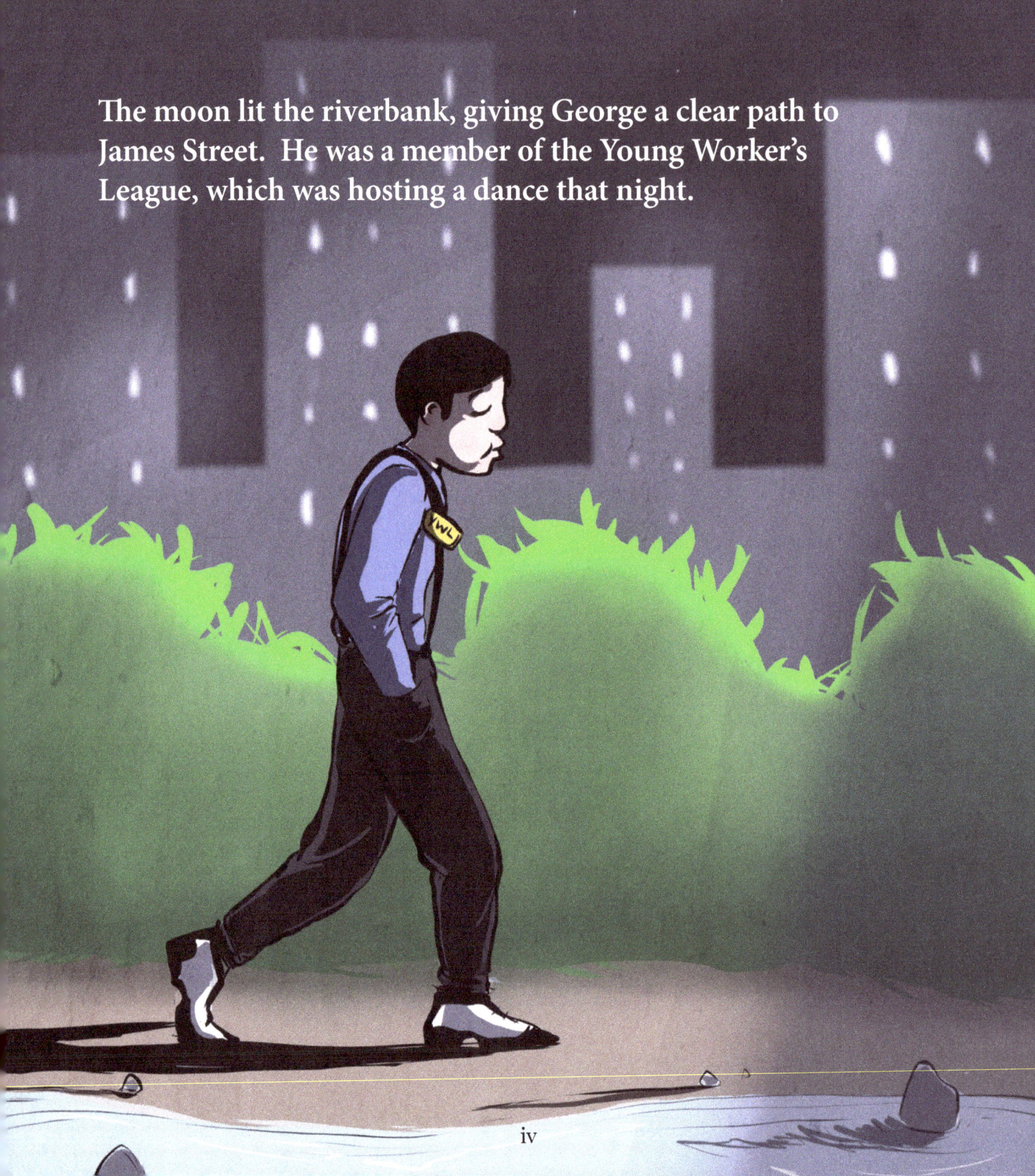

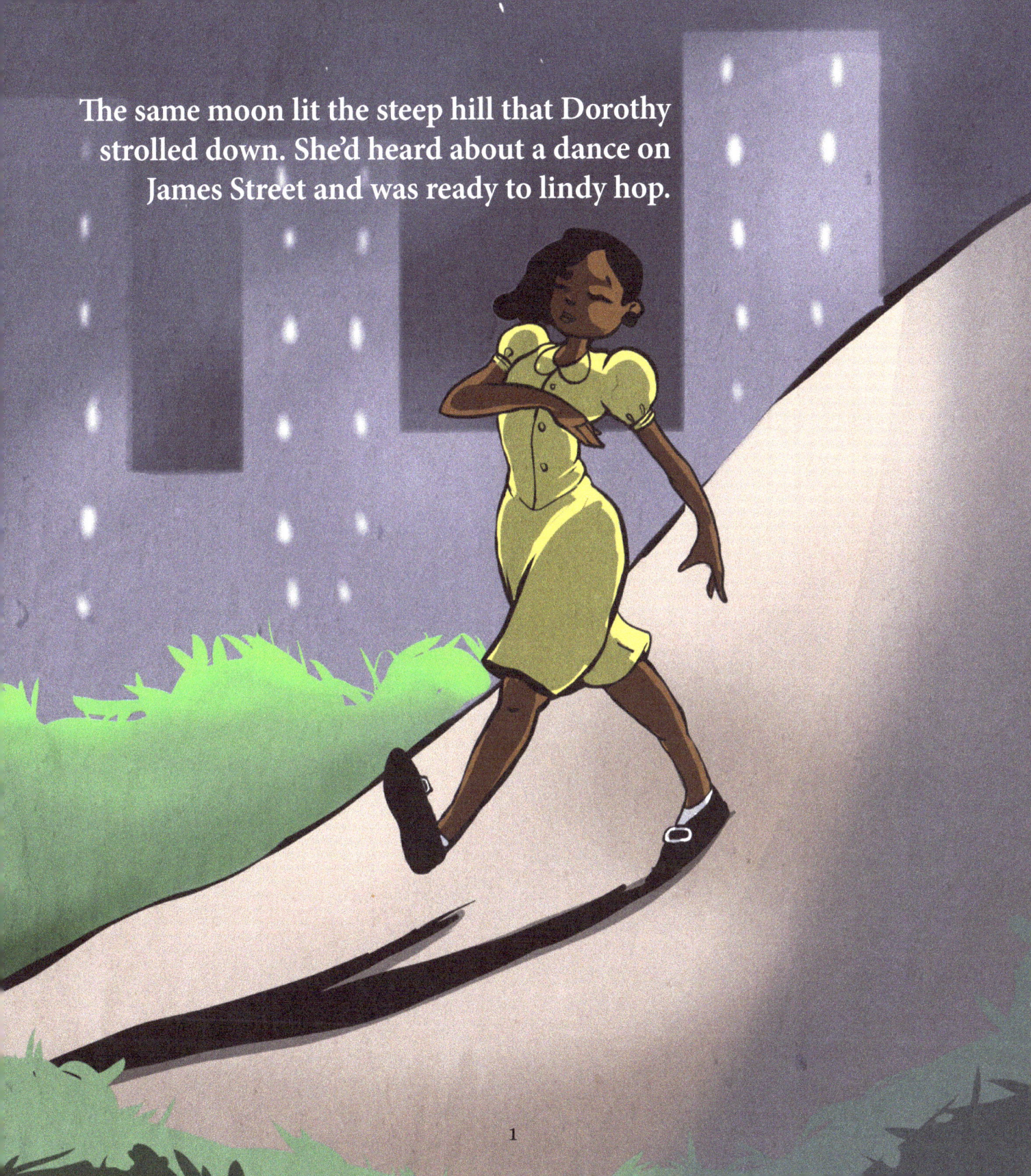

George picked up the pace as he heard a soft… *Rat a tat, rat a tat, rat a tat, tat.*

Dorothy heard it too and gave a twirl, testing out her new dress…
Rat a tat, rat a tat, rat a tat, tat.

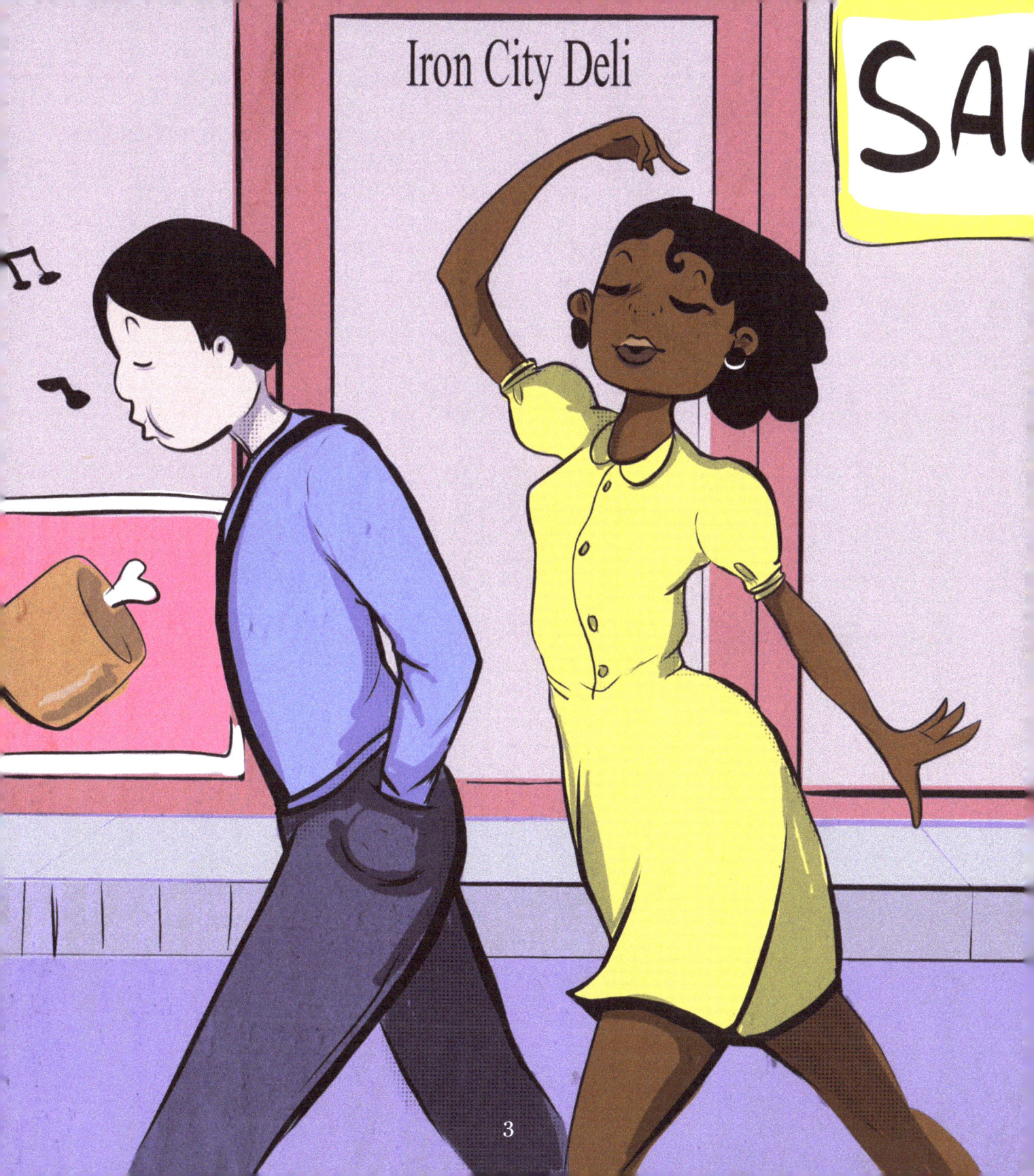

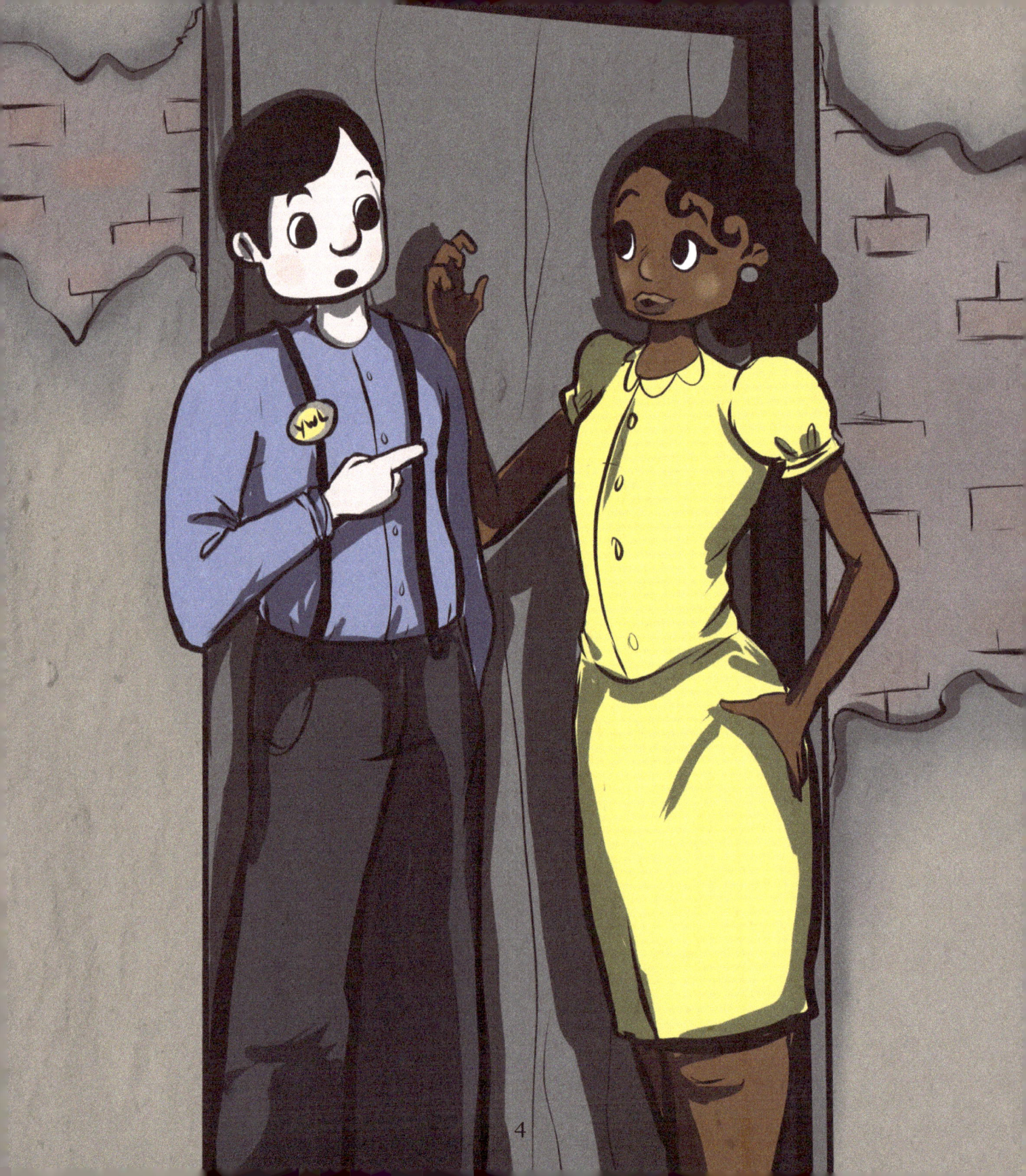

Two hands reached for the door of the dance hall. George pulled back, hoping the darkness would hide his burning cheeks.

"I'm Dorothy. Do you have a dance partner?" she asked.

"Do I need one?" George shrugged.

Dorothy laughed and held open the door. "ALL the best dances have partners," she said.

"Well in that case, would you like to dance?" he asked.

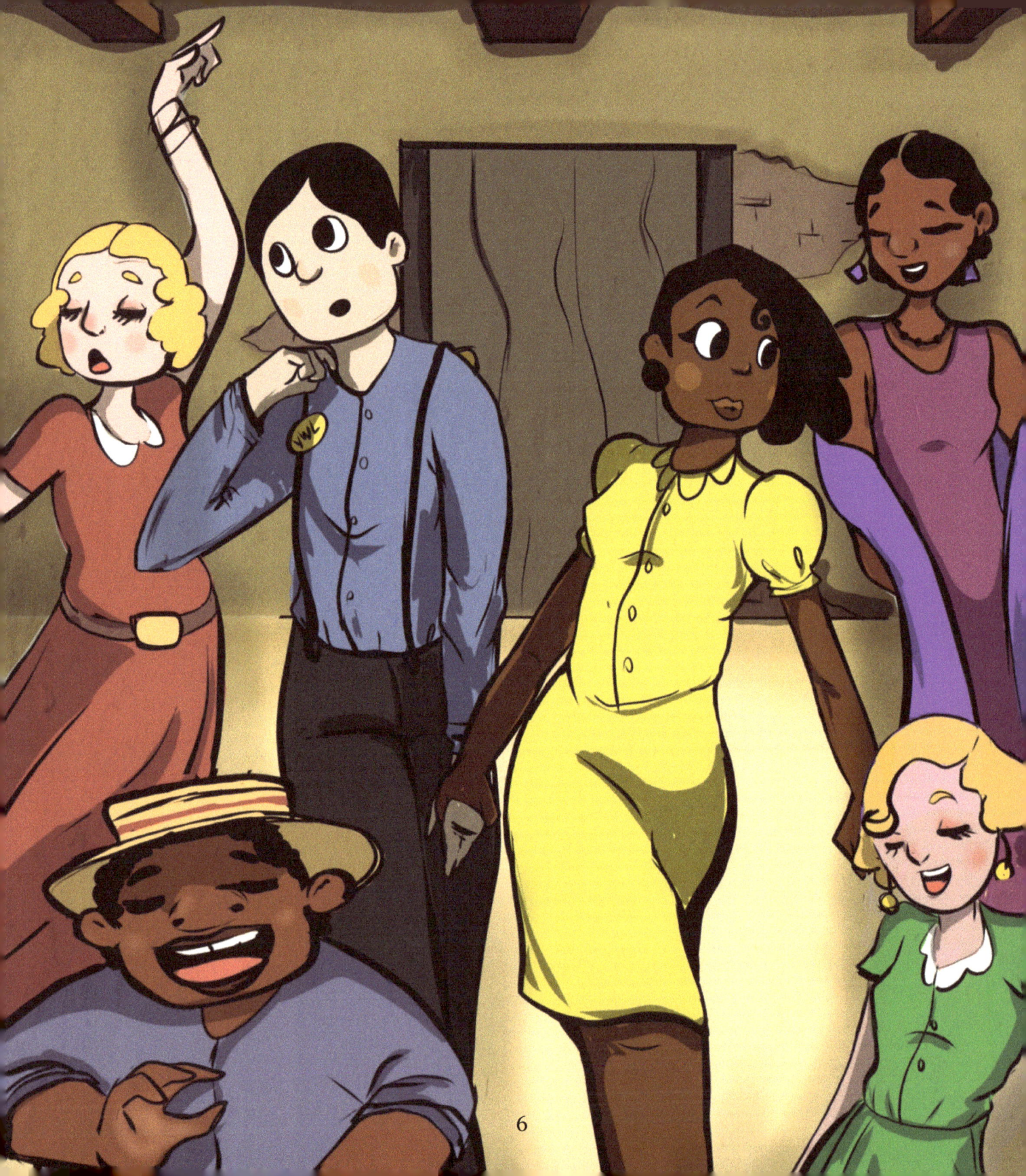

Dorothy grabbed George's hand and pulled him into the crowd. George hadn't realized how many kids would be there. It was packed, wall to wall. Everyone they passed smiled and waved at Dorothy. People stopped dancing to say hello to her.

George pulled at his shirt collar, surprised he'd agreed to lindy hop with someone so popular. He was going to make a fool out of himself at his first dance. He tried to wipe his sweaty palms on his pants as casually as he could.

Dorothy dragged him to the middle of the floor. "Are you ready?"

"Umm…"

She flashed him a wide smile. "We can watch the other kids for a while if you need a minute."

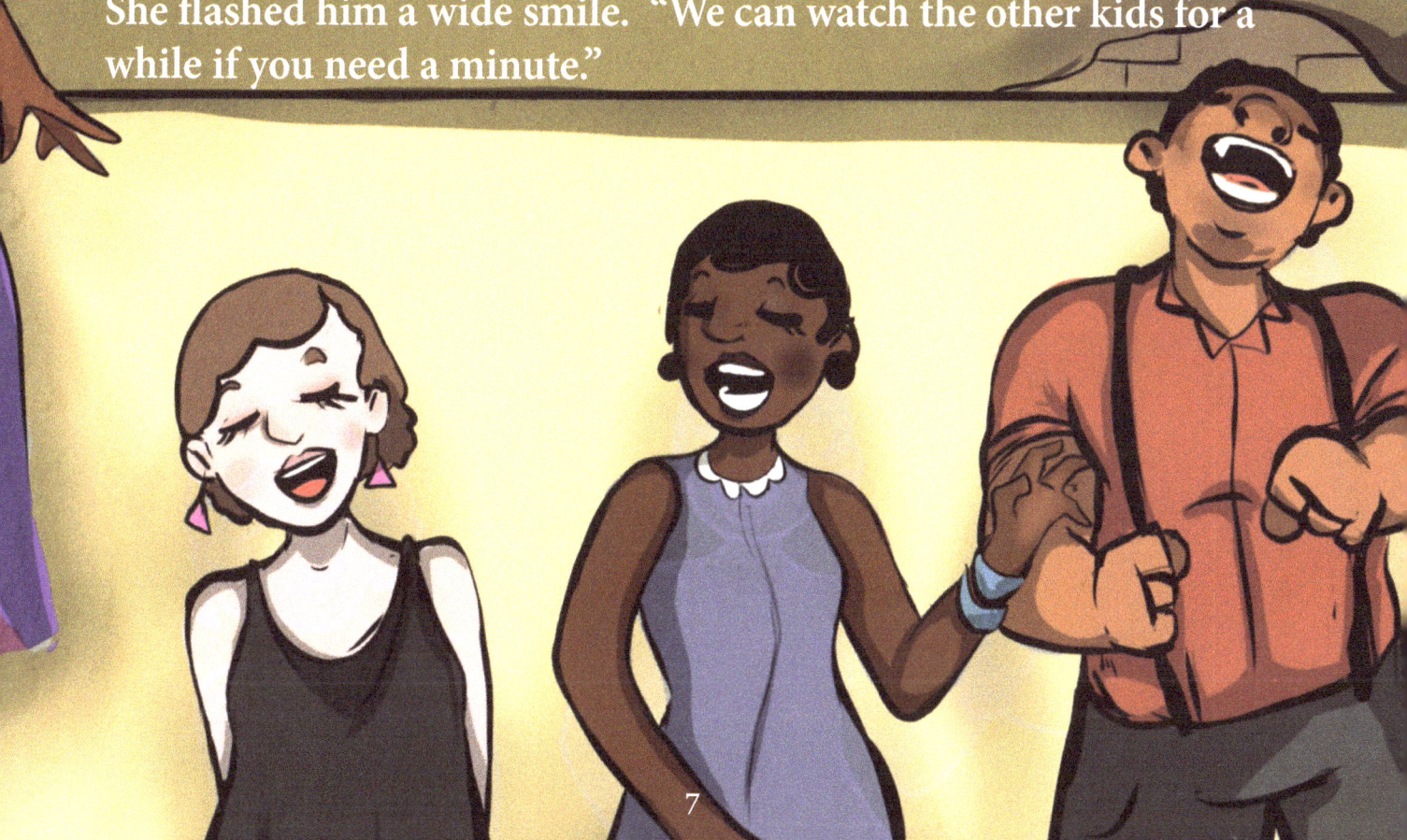

George nodded. It was getting easier to understand why everyone seemed to like Dorothy. Her confidence was uplifting, and she was clearly kind.

He took a deep breath. He'd lindy hopped a few times, but just to amuse his little sister and never in front of a crowd. He needed to pay attention to what was happening on the dance floor so he didn't screw this up.

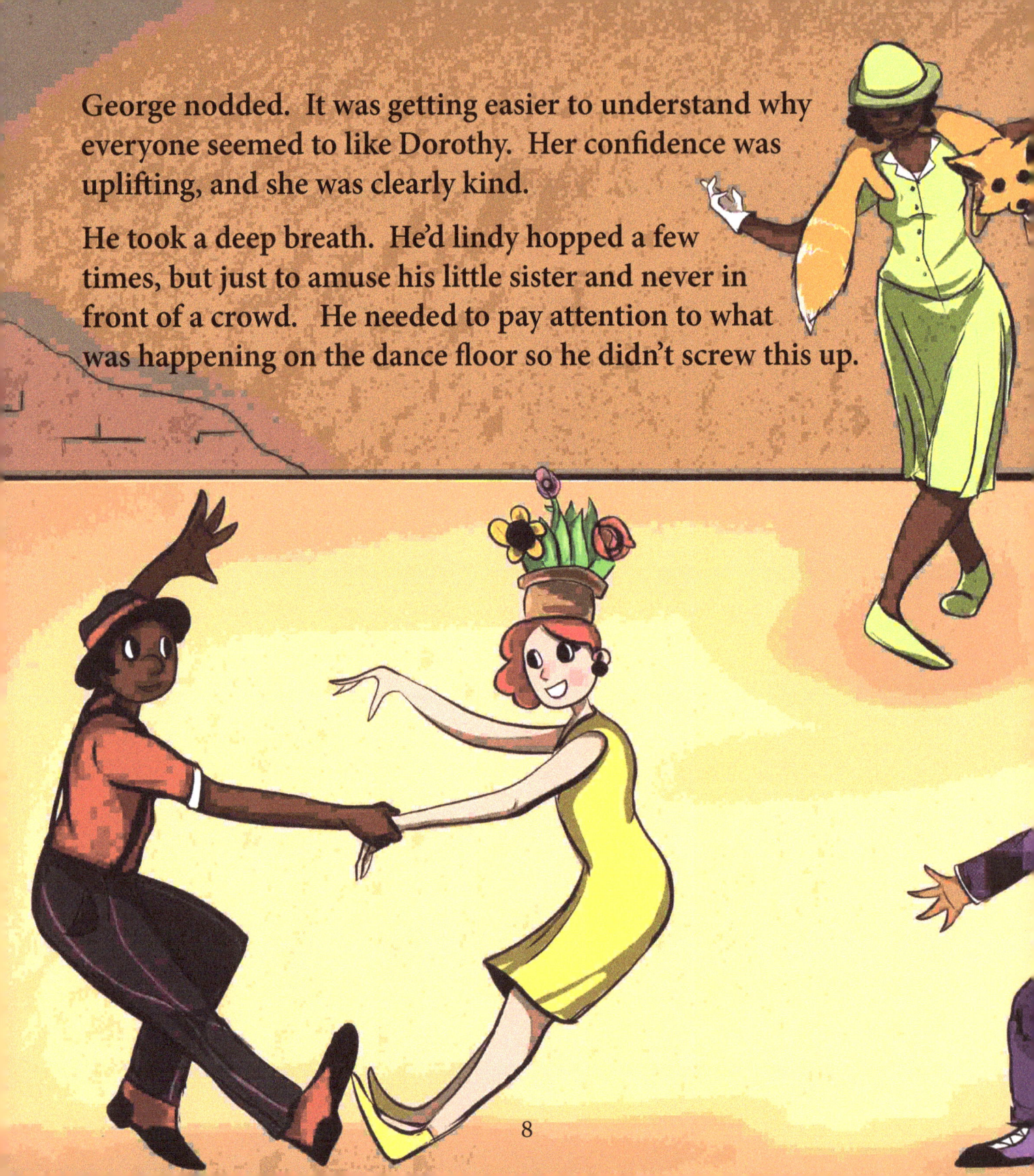

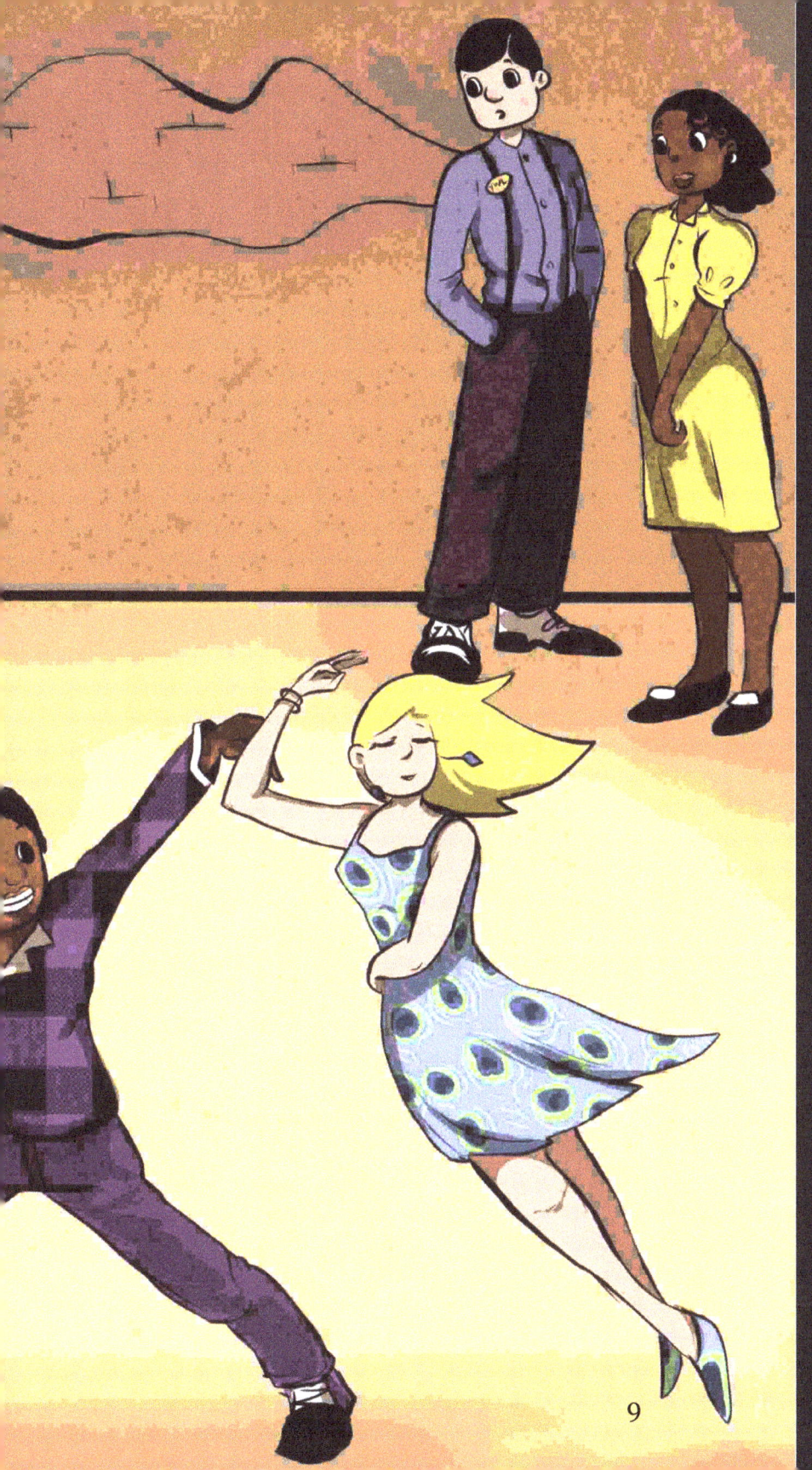

The kids all had style. Shined shoes and suit jackets. Brimmed hats and twisting skirts. Wait, did that girl have a fox around her neck? Did that one have a flower pot on her head? A boy flew by who looked like a checkerboard. He was twirling a girl who looked like a peacock. He couldn't wait to tell his little sister about these outfits, the moves, the music. That is, if he could trust her not to snitch to Mom and Dad.

"How do people afford these fancy clothes?" George asked earnestly.

"My Mamma made mine from a flour bag," Dorothy gave another spin. "And I bet a lot of the dresses in here are made from feedbags"

"Feedbags?" George got distracted imagining farm animals in fancy dresses.

"Enough gawking, let's dance!" Dorothy yelled over the music into George's ear.

Snake hips, Suzie Q, Shim-Sham. A ring fling, a ring fling, a ring a fling, ZING.

George closed his eyes and listened to the beat.

A boom, a bam, a boom boom BAM.

"Now we got it! Ready to lift… just don't drop me!" Dorothy said.

George gulped and nodded.

Bend the knees, push up, FROG JUMP.

Rat a tat, rat a tat, rat a tat, tat.

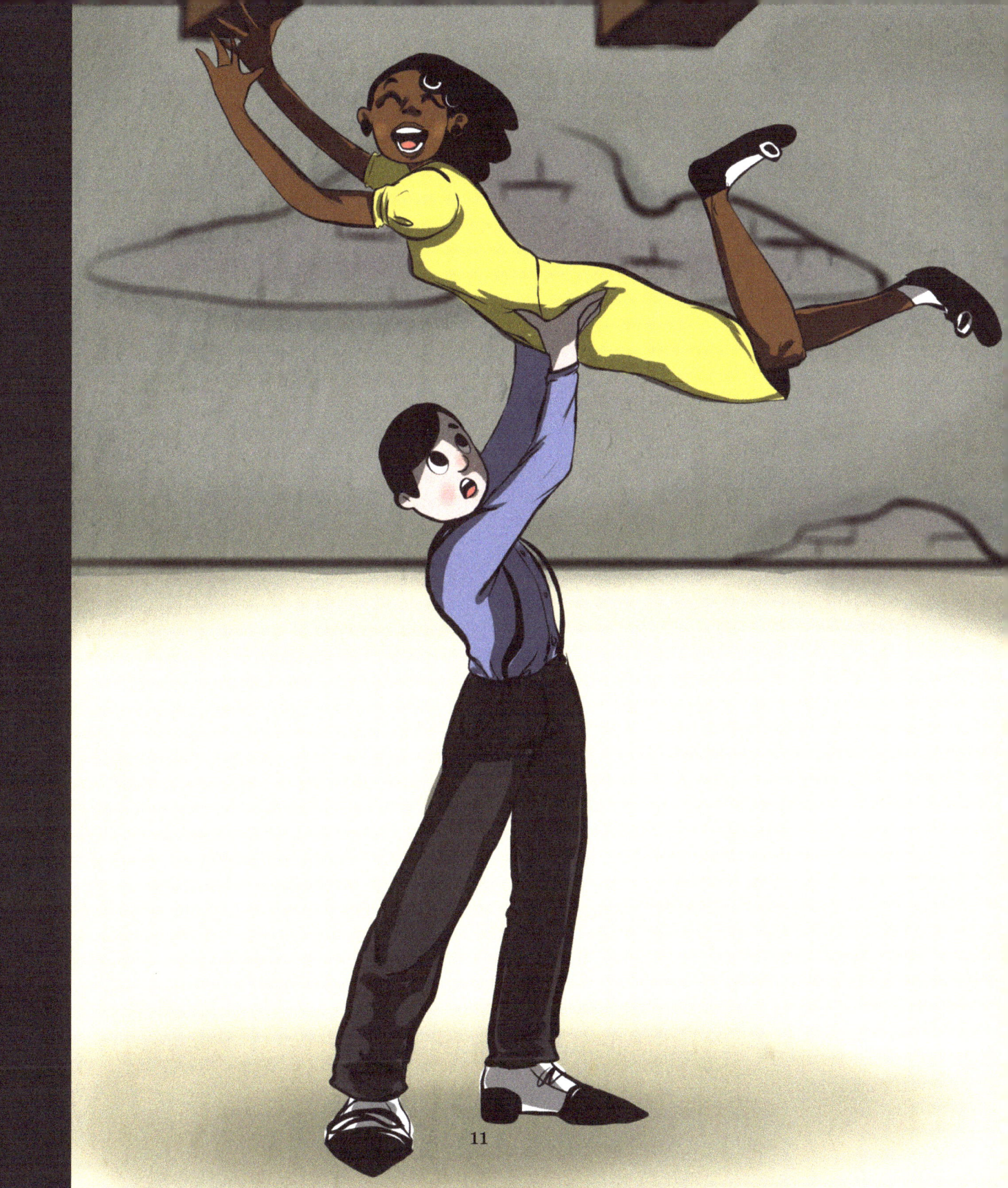

Dorothy was smiling and laughing when she landed back on the ground. "You're getting the hang of it now. Want to take a break and grab some water?"

George nodded and they headed to the back.

"How come I haven't seen you around before now? Everyone seems to know you."

Dorothy narrowed her eyes at him, "We aren't exactly allowed to hangout in the same places, are we?"

"Oh, right." George tapped his foot. He put his hands in his pockets then took them out again, suddenly unsure of what to do with them. He wished he hadn't asked Dorothy such a foolish question.

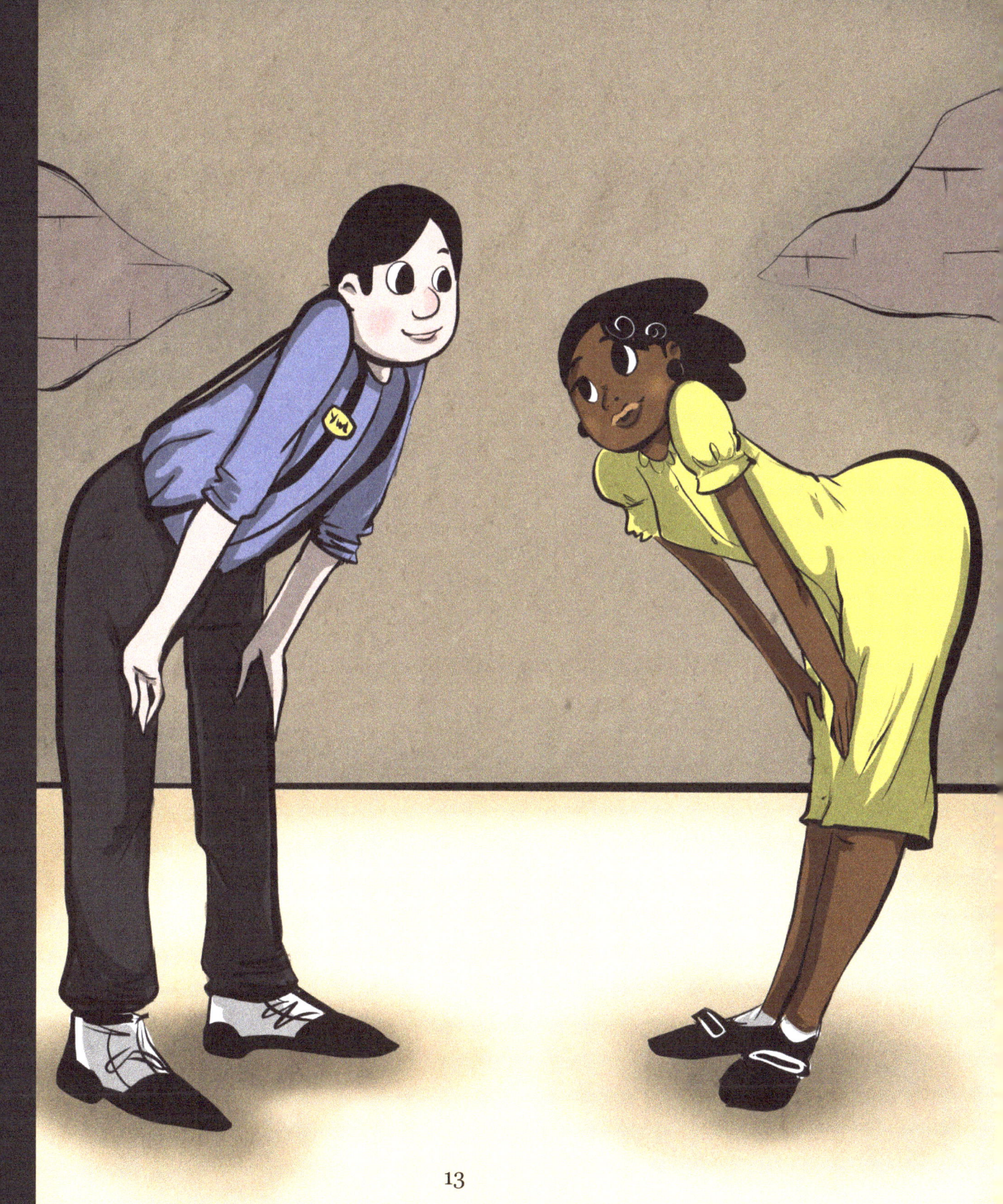

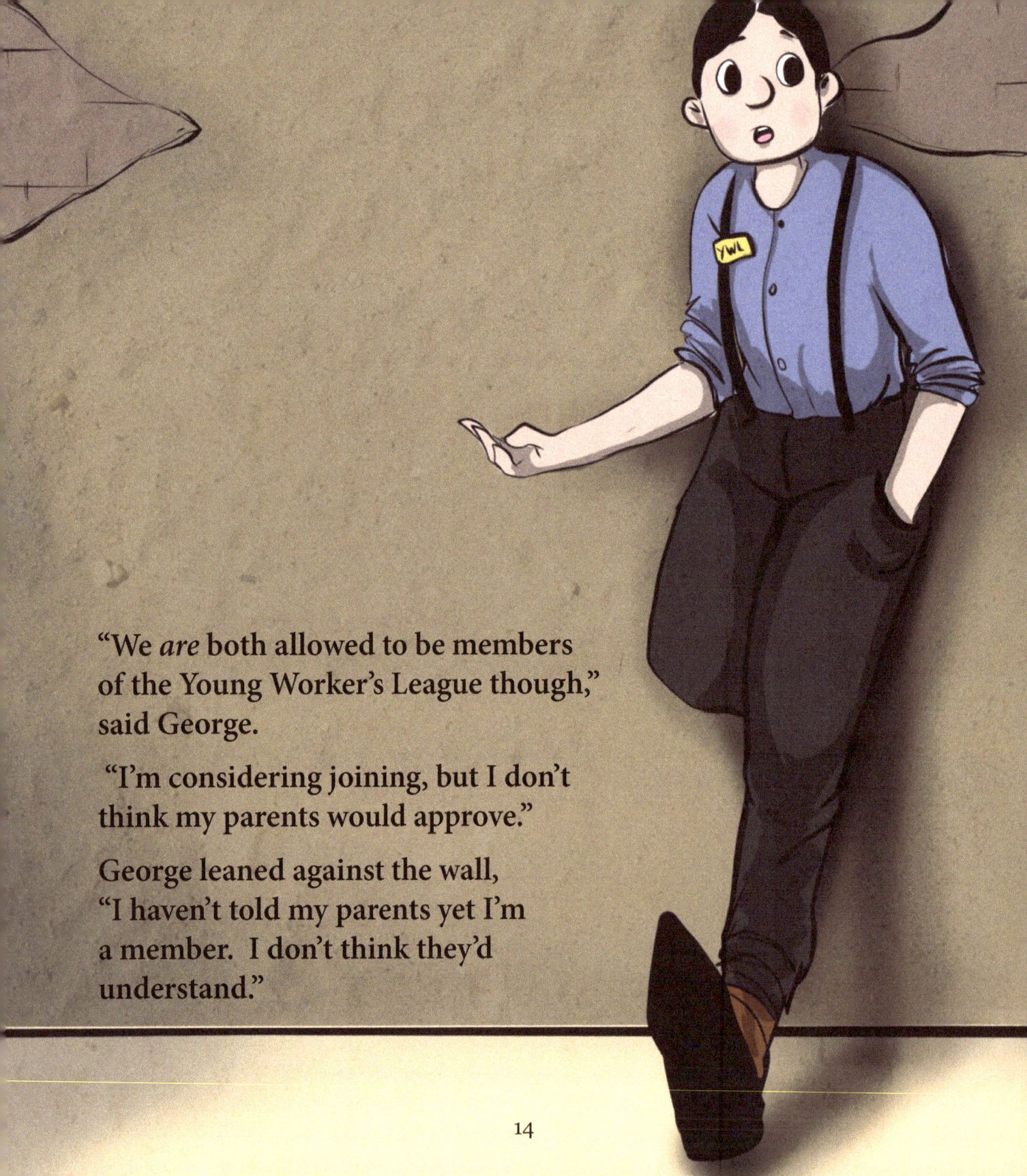

"We *are* both allowed to be members of the Young Worker's League though," said George.

"I'm considering joining, but I don't think my parents would approve."

George leaned against the wall, "I haven't told my parents yet I'm a member. I don't think they'd understand."

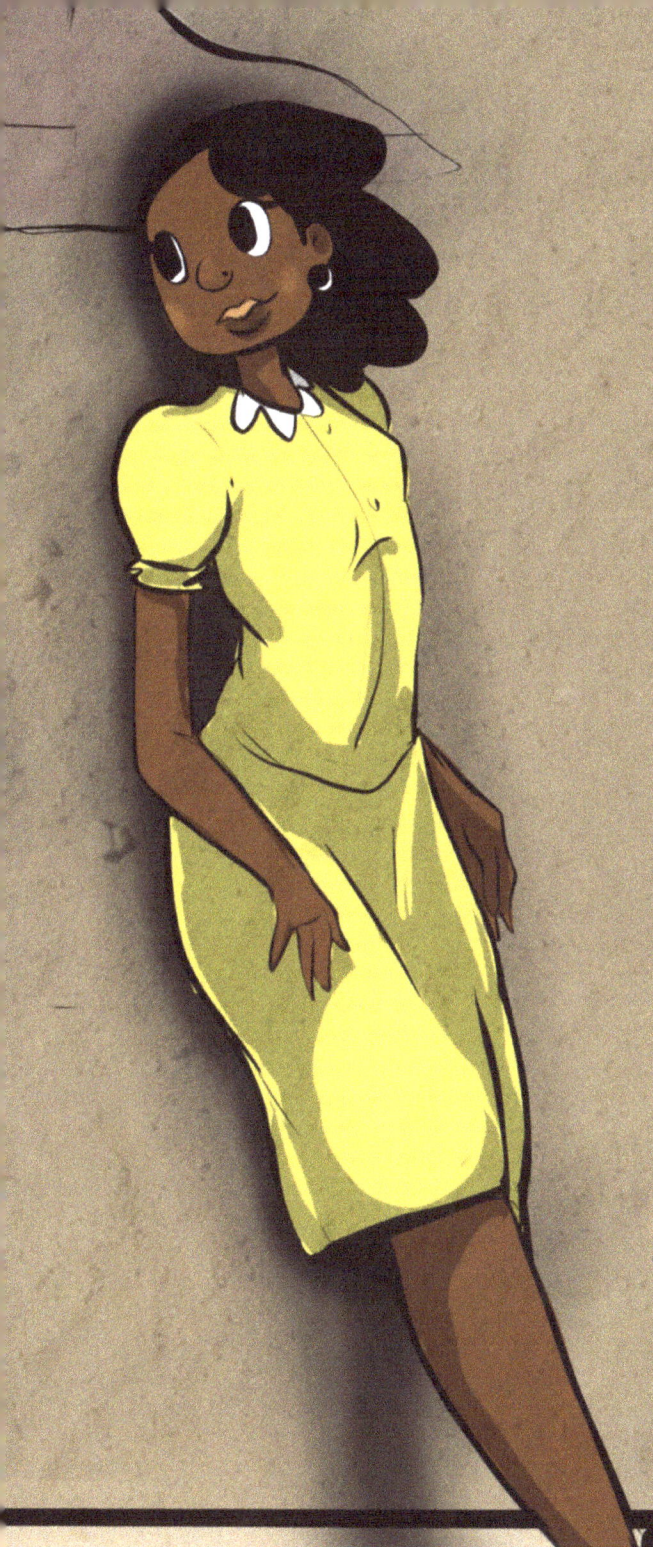

"What would they think of you dancing with *me*?"

George ran his hand through his hair and thought about it. "They probably wouldn't understand that, either."

"The world is changing, whether our parents like it or not."

"You're such a good dancer. You ever think about dancing in a contest?" said George.

"My dream is to go to New York one day and dance at the Savoy Ballroom."

"Wow, all the way to New York. I've never even been across the Allegheny river." George gestured back to the dance floor. "Should we try again? I think I'm getting better."

Dorothy winked at him. "You have a good teacher."

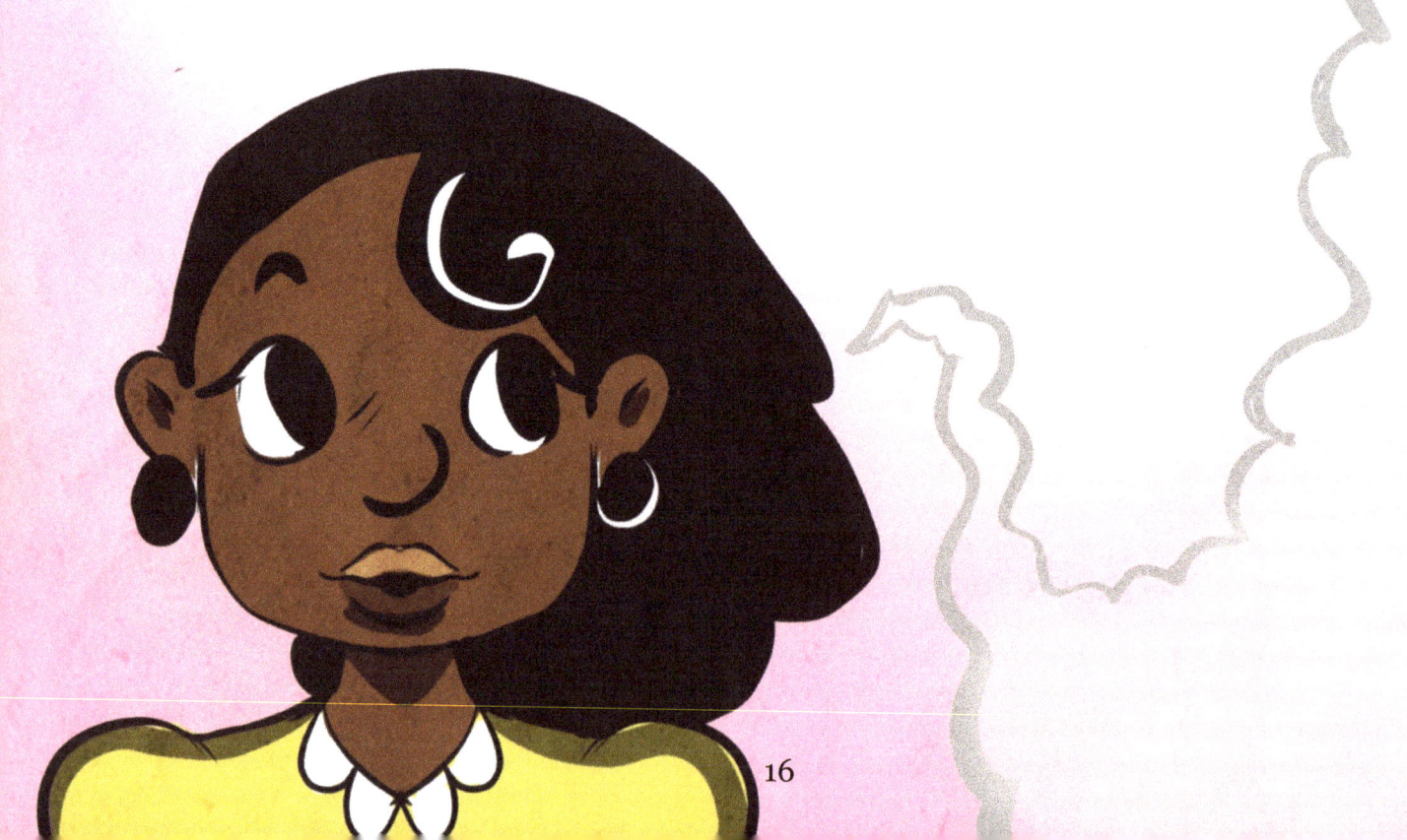

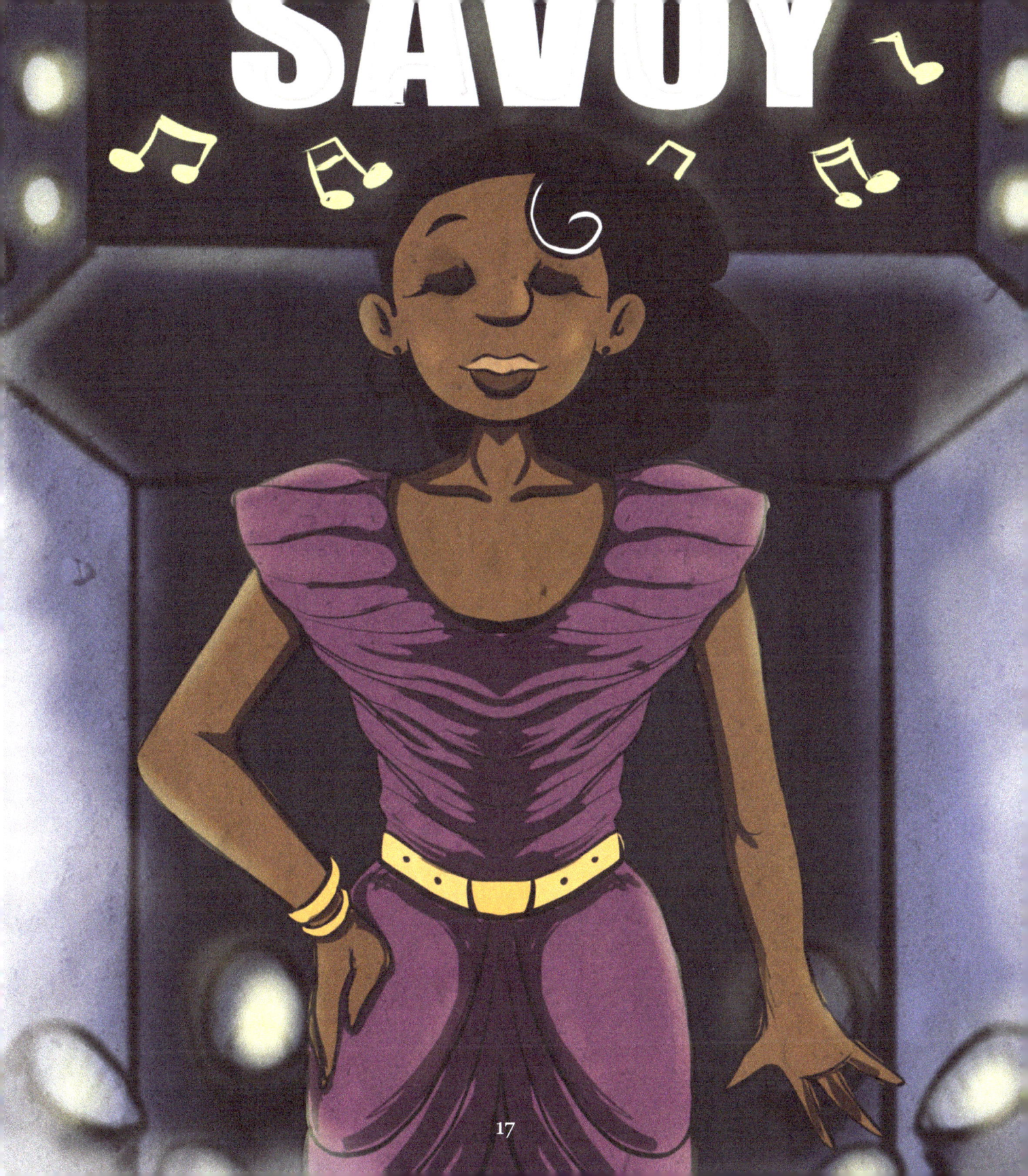

An hour later a ring of kids gathered around Dorothy and George as they flew across the floor. Soon they were the only two dancing, with the others cheering them on. The kids clapped and stomped their feet to the music. Dorothy's confidence was contagious and George was throwing her higher and jumping faster.

George felt light and free as he twisted and twirled his way across the room.

Rat a tat, rat a tat, rat a tat, tat…Hacksaw. Hip Lift. Peel Away. BOOM. Slide Drag Dig. BAM BAM BAM.

Around the world AND Whip.

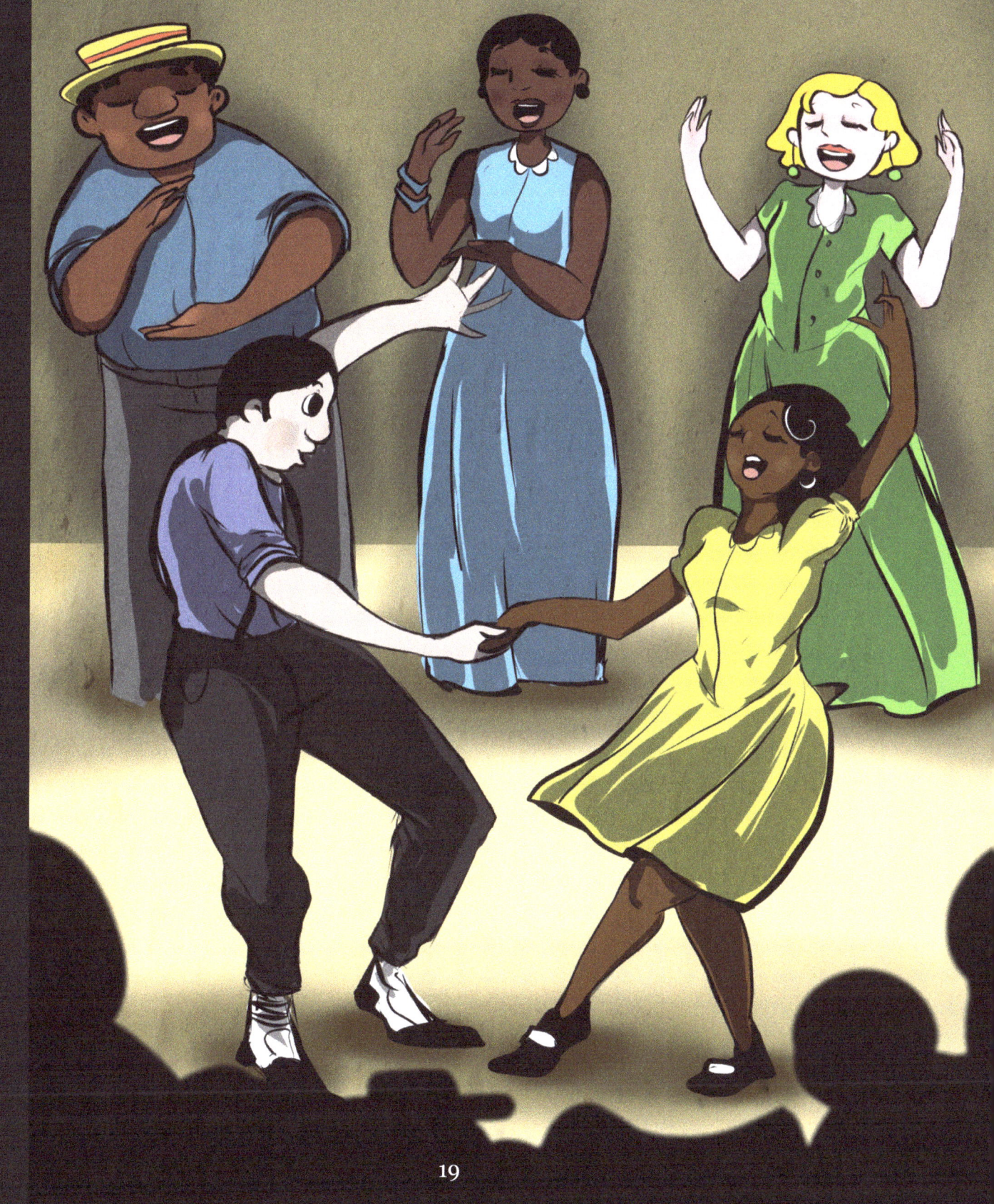

Suddenly there came a BANG. Police officers filled the doorway to the dance hall. The officer in front pointed right at Dorothy and George.

"This dance is being shut down due to blacks and whites dancing together!" he bellowed. George looked over at Dorothy.

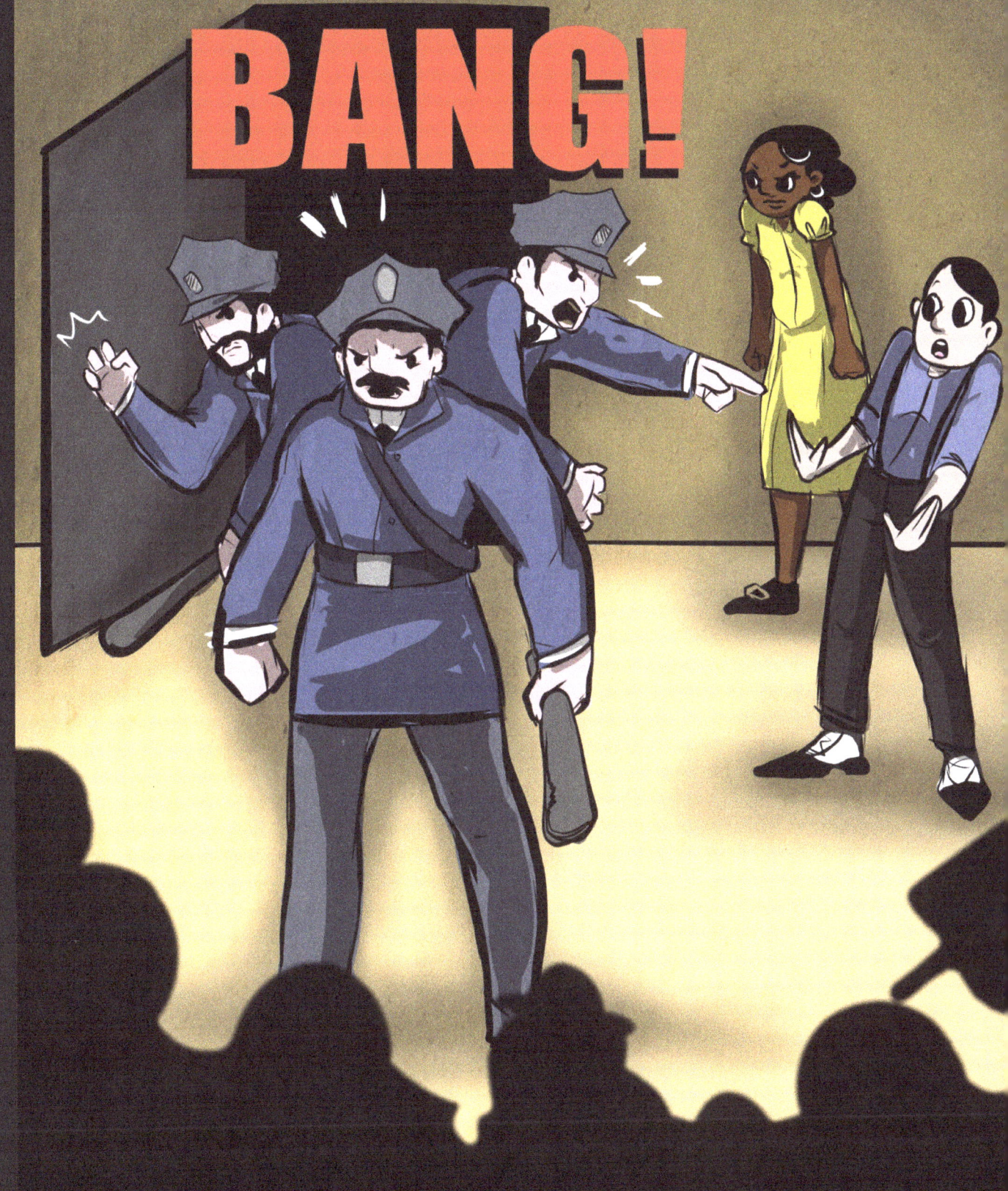

Officers began knocking kids over and shoving them against the wall. Some were carrying clubs. George saw an officer use his club to bash a kid in the back of the knees. The kid screamed and toppled over. George froze. He was used to the police helping kids cross the street outside his school, not attacking them. These police officers were twice the size as most of the kids at the dance.

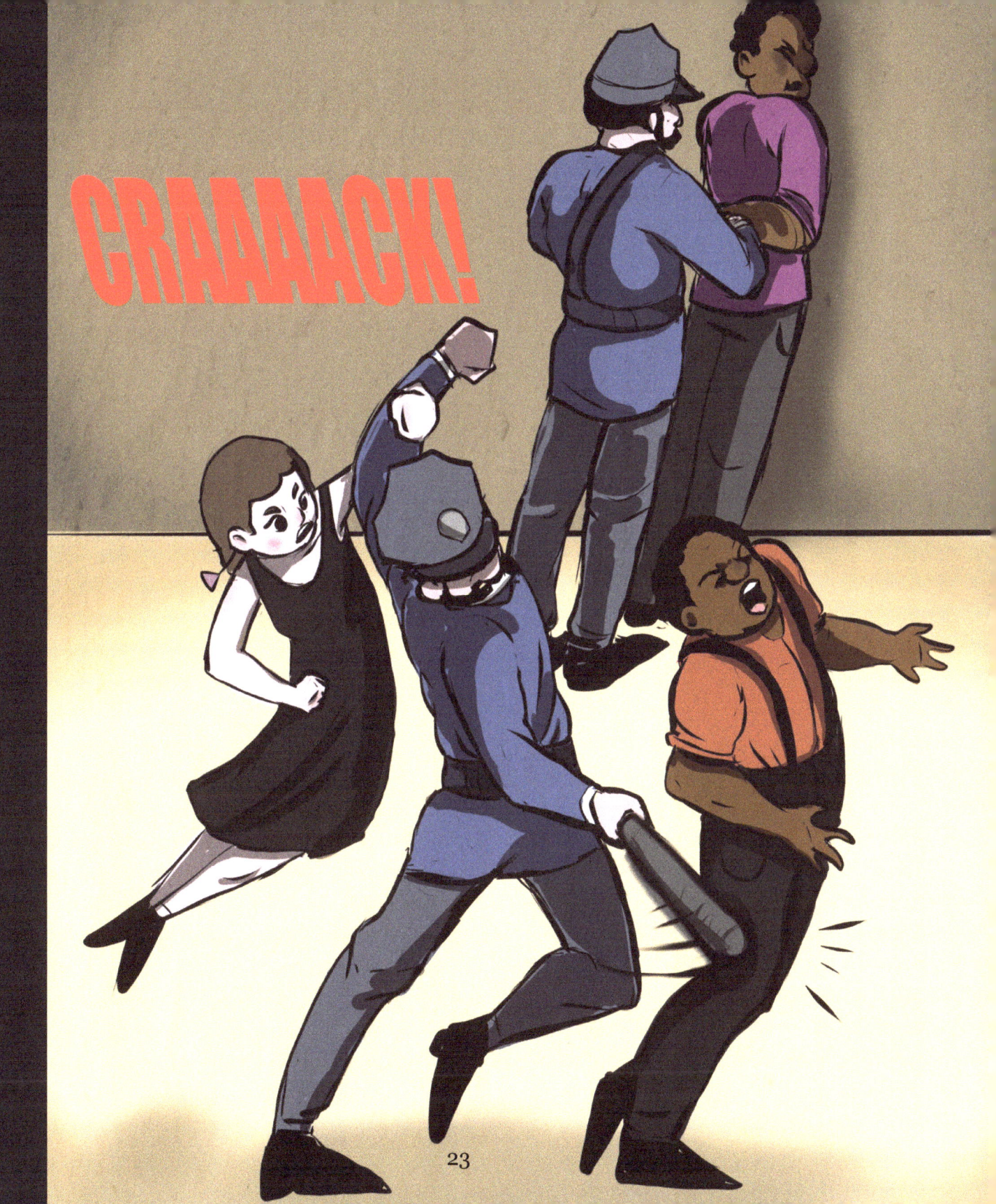

"RUN!" came a voice from the back. Kids began to scatter. Dorothy grabbed George's hand again and pulled him out the back door.

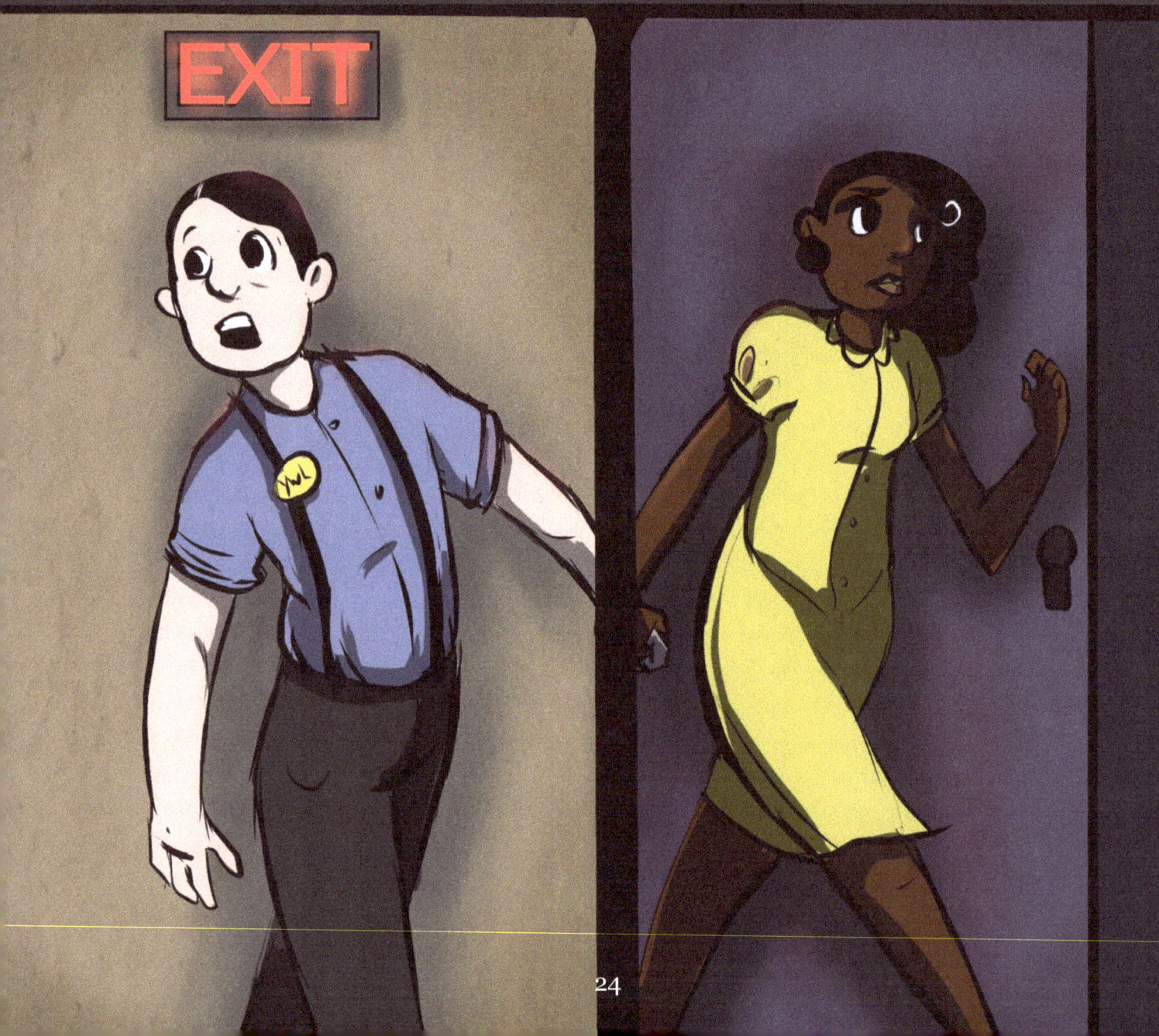

Thump, thump, thump, went their feet down James street. They got a few blocks away and hid low behind some bushes. They saw a few more kids run past them. One had blood dripping down his face. Another was limping.

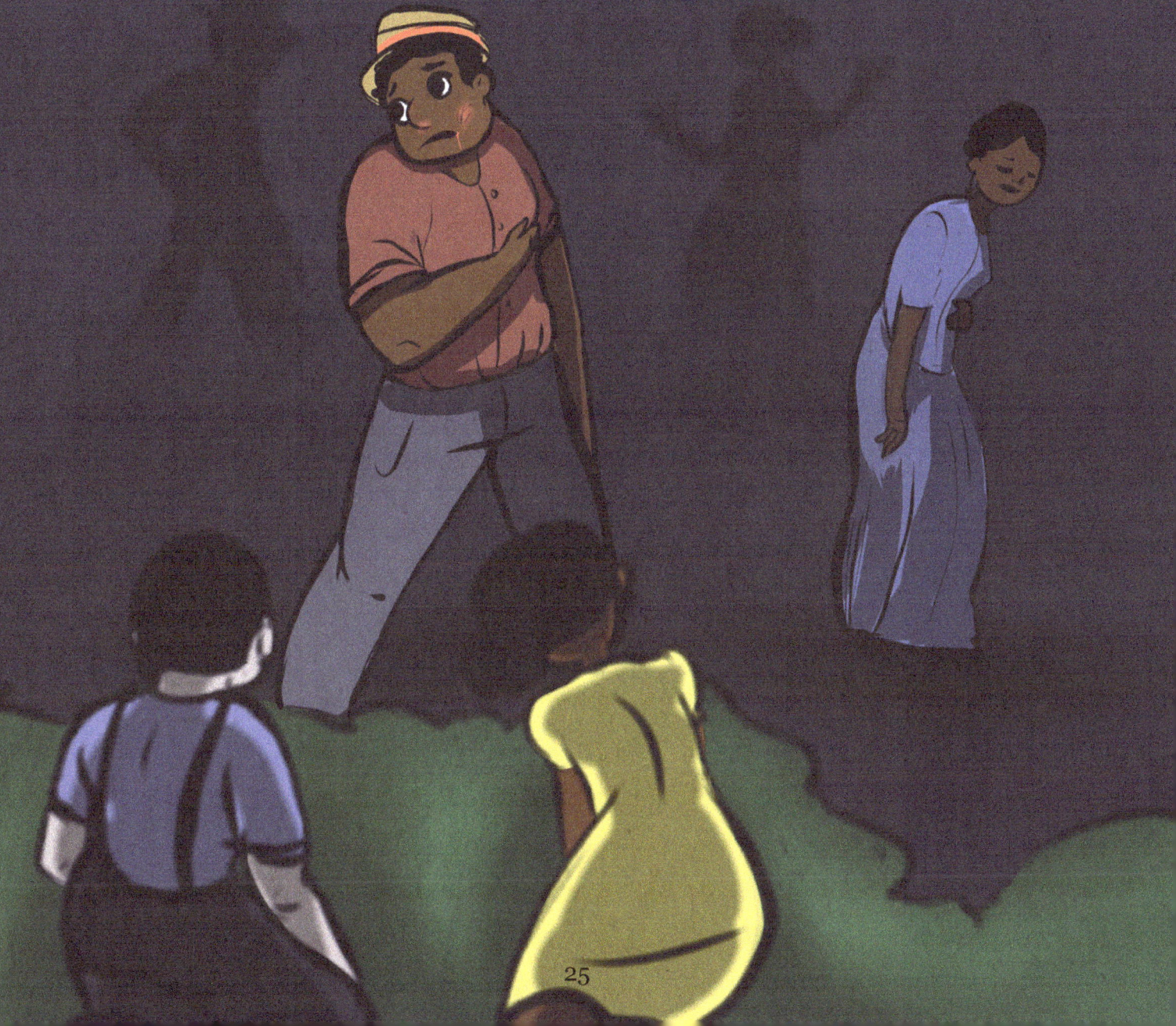

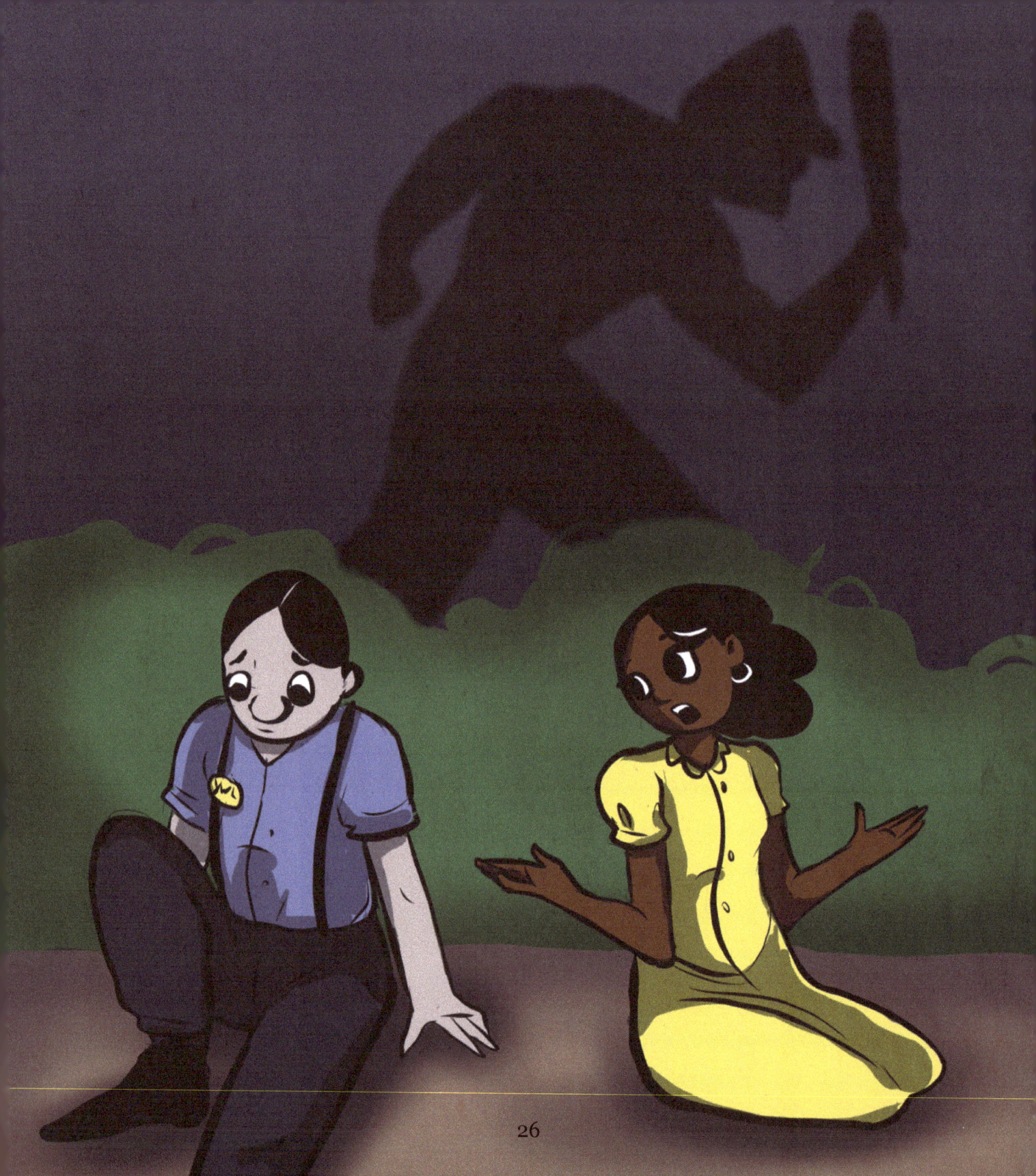

"This isn't right," George said. He looked down at his feet. He felt afraid and ashamed.

"You don't have to tell me, this is a regular part of my life." Dorothy ducked lower as an officer ran by.

"Well, it shouldn't be."

"What are you going to do about it?"

"What do you mean?"

"You said *it isn't right*. So, what are you going to do about it?"

"I-I-I- don't know… the police shut it down… what else *can* we do?"

"We can't let them stop us from dancing. I have an idea," said Dorothy. "The police are less likely to bother you than me. Run down the side streets and grab all the kids you can find. Tell them to come to my house at the top of the hill."

Before George could respond Dorothy was gone. His shoulders sank as he slowly headed back towards the main road. He'd never been confronted by the police before and his hands trembled.

George considered his options. He could go home and pretend this night never happened. He thought of the police officers as they raised their clubs to innocent kids. No, he'd never forget this night.

He could go home and explain what had happened to his parents, maybe they would know the right thing to do. There were a few problems with this plan. Firstly, his parents thought he was staying over at his friends Ricky's, they didn't even know he was at a dance. And secondly, he'd never heard his parents talk about segregation.

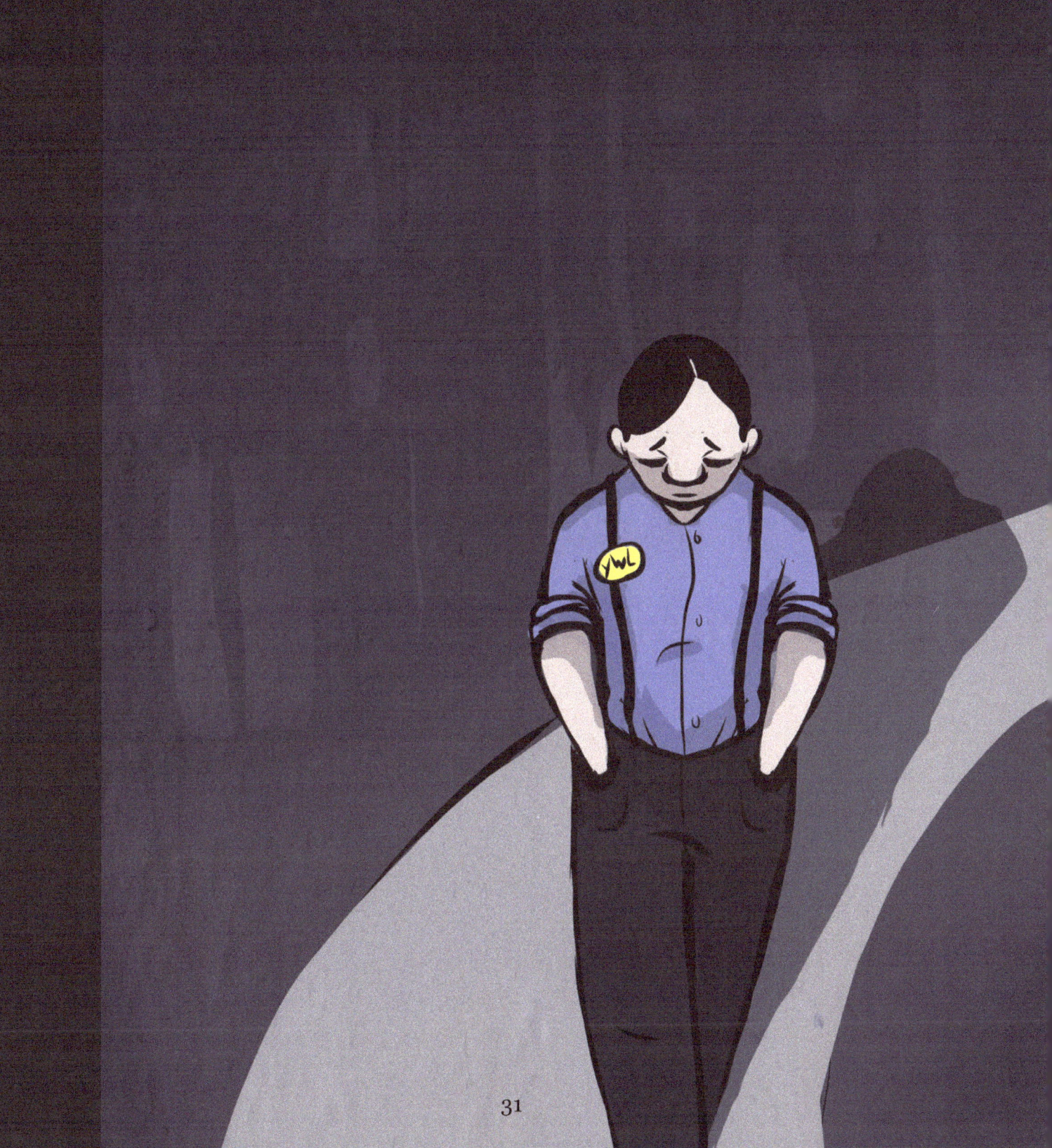

George couldn't remember a time in his whole life that he saw his parents interacting with a Black person unless that person was a worker. Their church, the stores they shopped at, their school… it was all white people. He was going to need to talk to his parents about segregation, but he didn't have time to go home and do that just then, he needed to act. Now.

He could try going to the police and reasoning with them himself. What would he say? "You need to stop enforcing a bad law?" George kicked the curb in frustration. No, no, no. That wasn't right either.

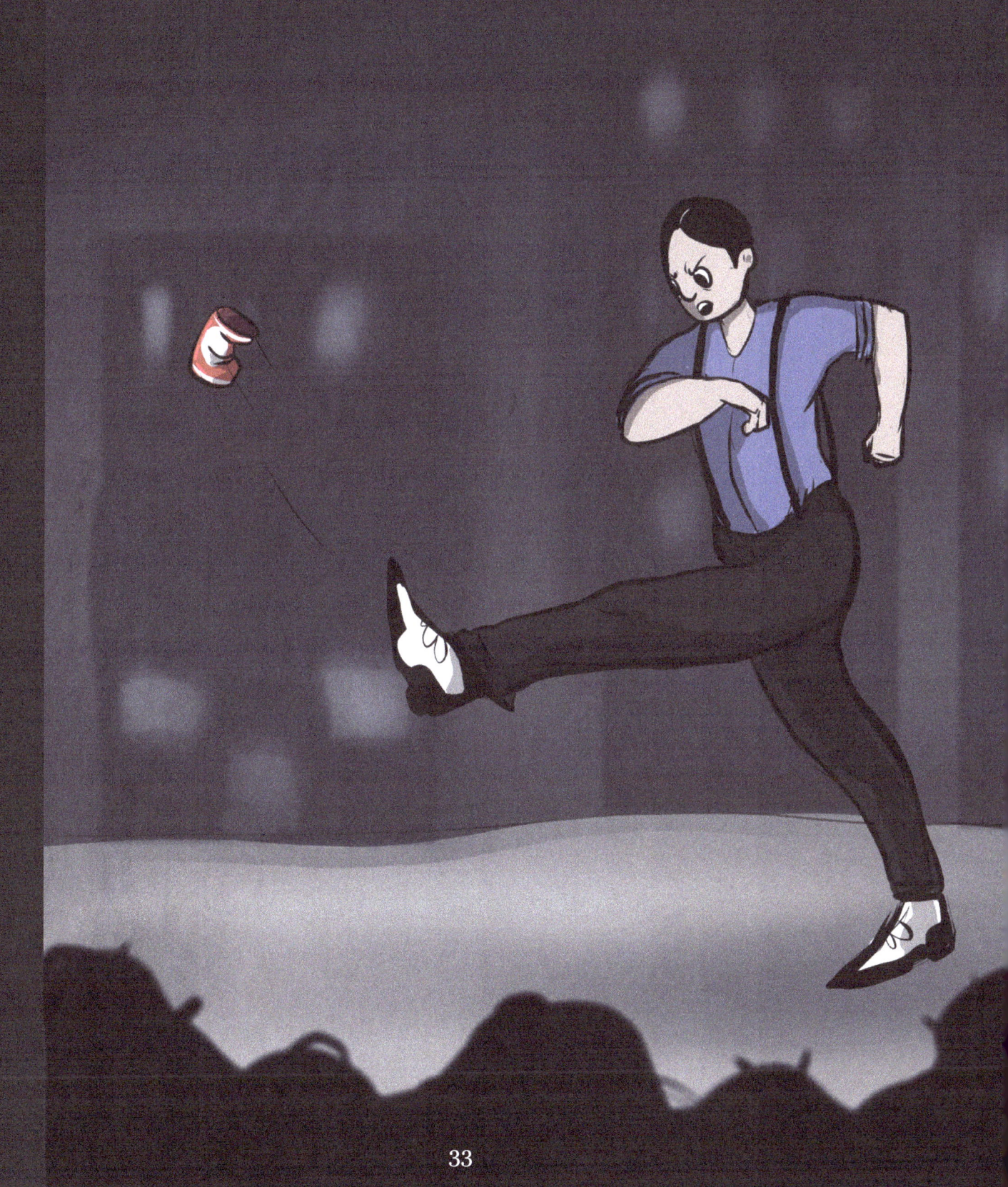

George froze as he saw a police officer running in his direction. He'd gotten in fights with neighborhood boys before and defended himself pretty well, but he never fought with a grown man. As fear pulsed through his body from his fingers down to his toes, the officer ran by him. George's cheeks burned red. If it had been Dorothy there on the corner and not him… What would have happened? He had been at the dance. He had been breaking the law by dancing with Dorothy. Why did the police officer run right past him?

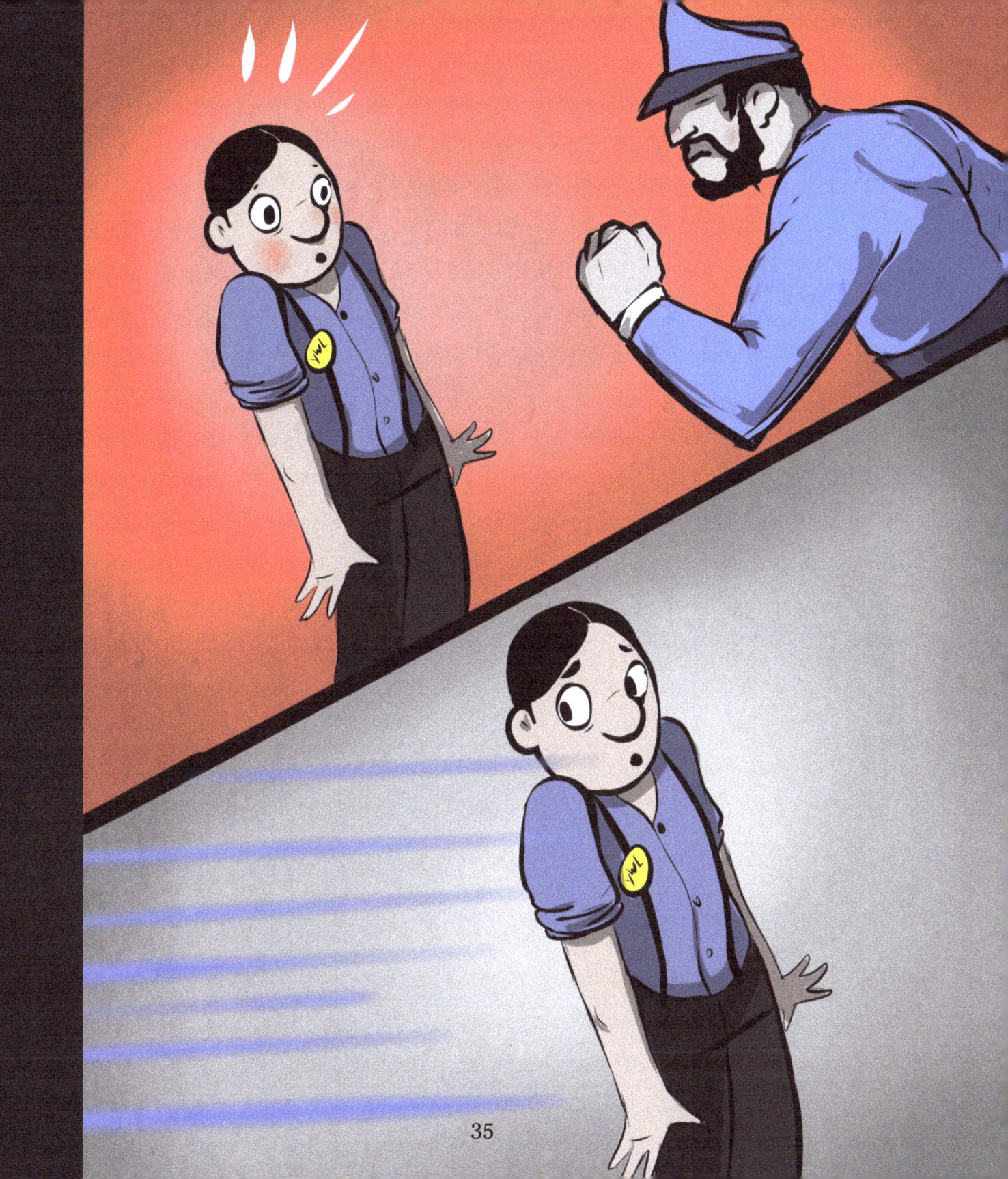

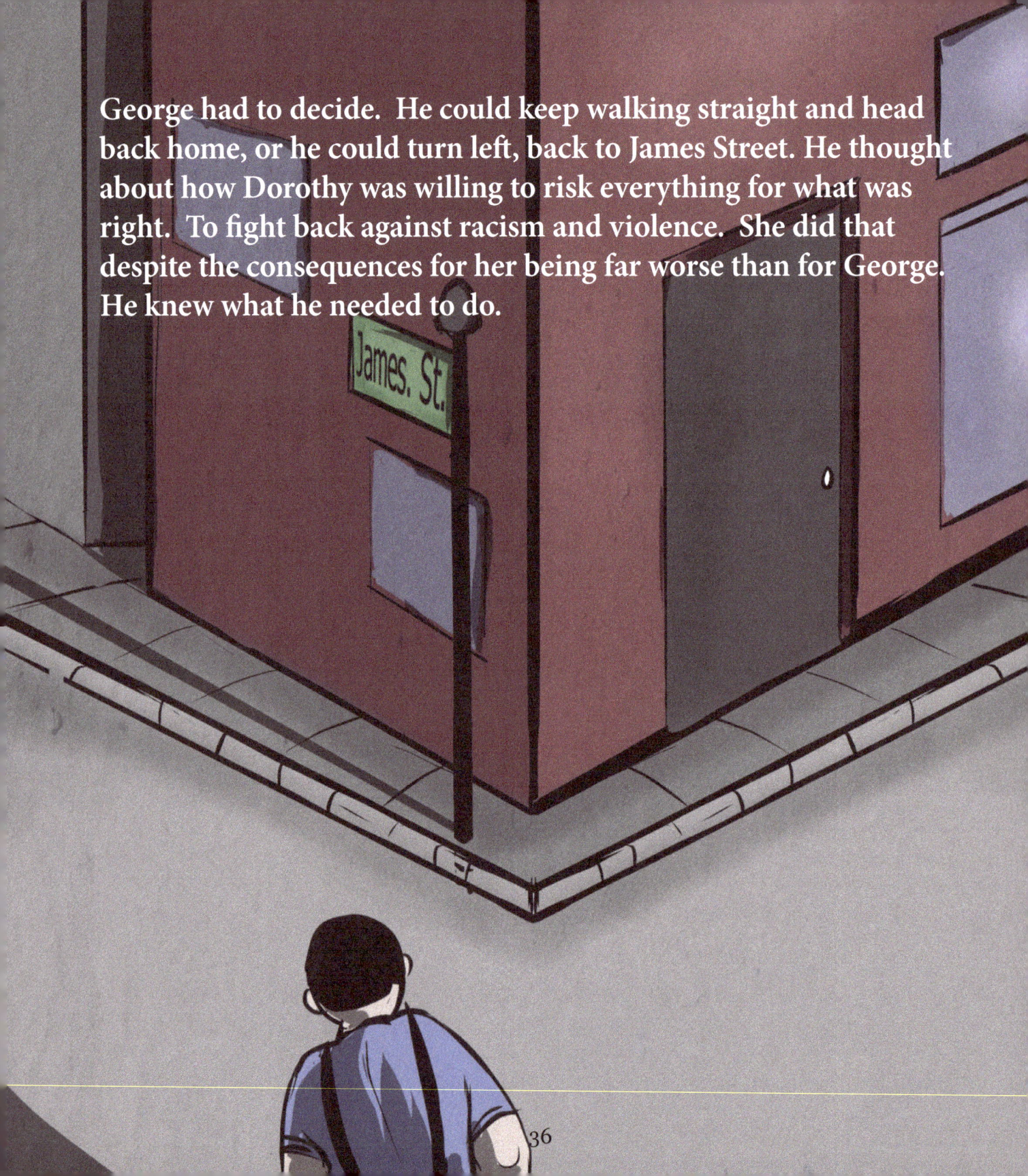

George had to decide. He could keep walking straight and head back home, or he could turn left, back to James Street. He thought about how Dorothy was willing to risk everything for what was right. To fight back against racism and violence. She did that despite the consequences for her being far worse than for George. He knew what he needed to do.

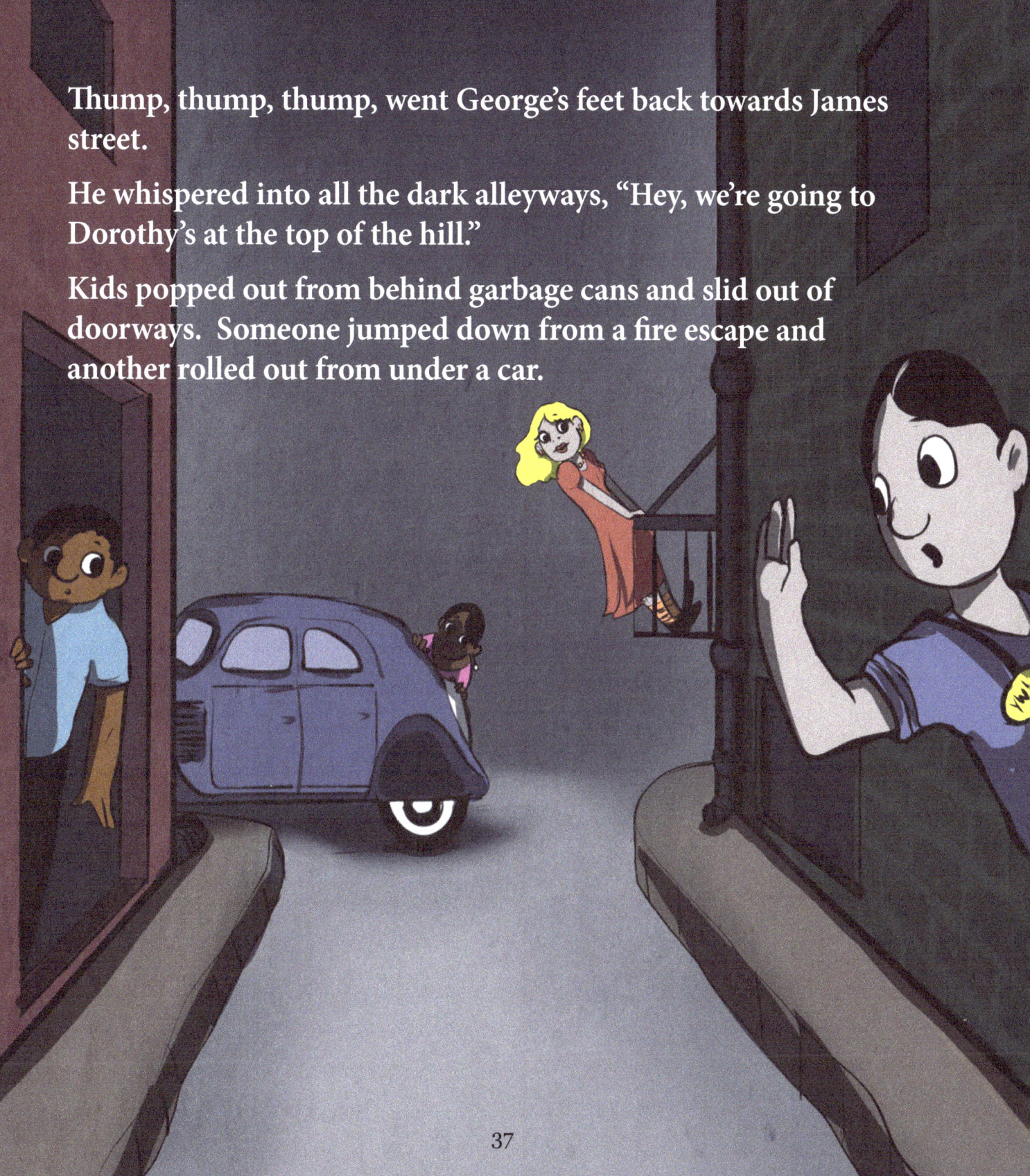

Thump, thump, thump, went George's feet back towards James street.

He whispered into all the dark alleyways, "Hey, we're going to Dorothy's at the top of the hill."

Kids popped out from behind garbage cans and slid out of doorways. Someone jumped down from a fire escape and another rolled out from under a car.

It wasn't long before George was making his way up the hill with a big group of kids. The moon had gone behind the clouds, giving them the shadows they needed.

And then they heard it…

Rat a tat, rat a tat, rat a tat, tat.

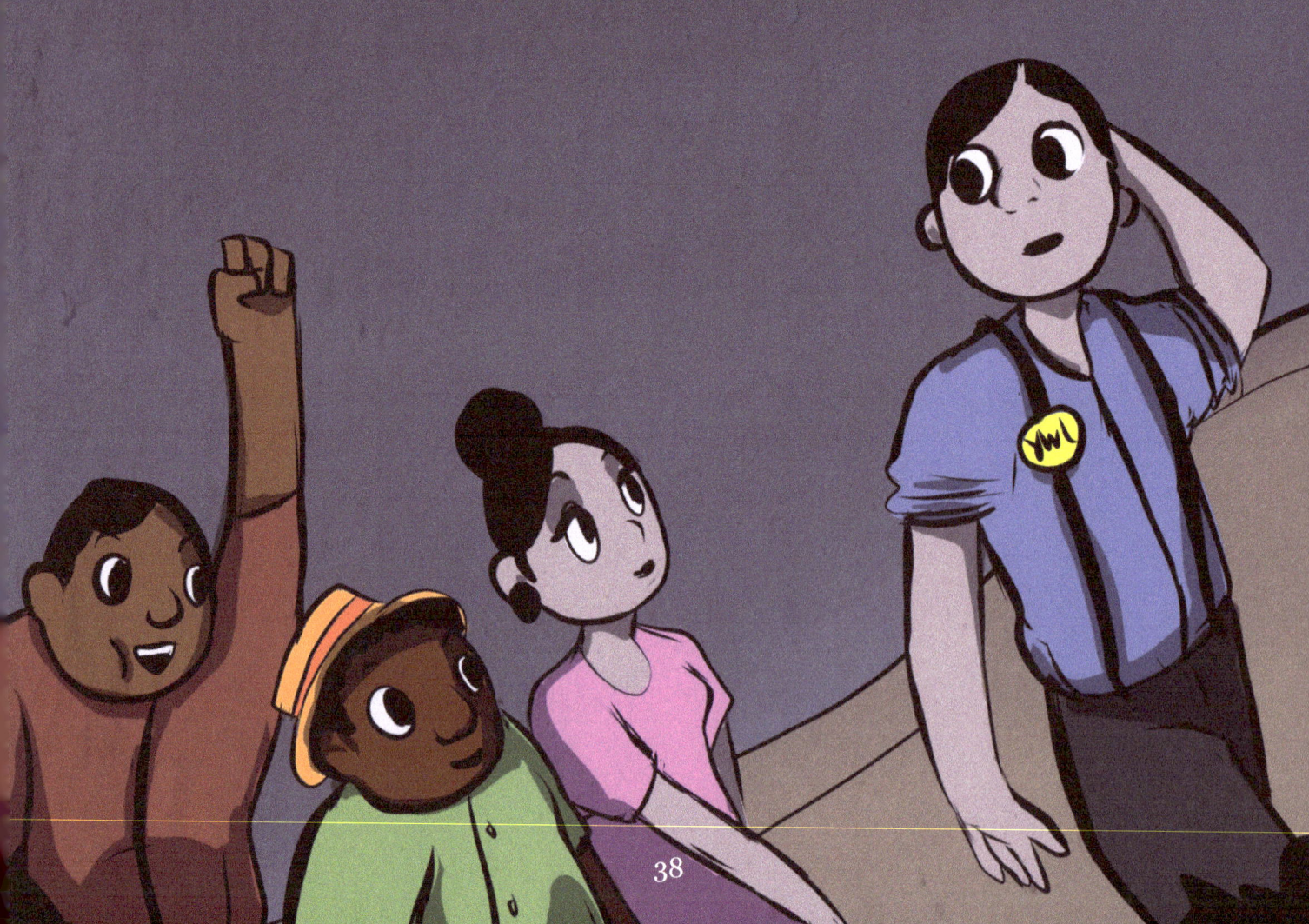

Dorothy burst onto the front porch just in time to see the pack of kids reaching the top of the hill. She smiled at the sight of them.

She put her hands on her hips and yelled out to the crowd, "We all know that separate isn't equal! We aren't going to let them stop us from dancing! Come inside, and let's HOP!"

The kids cheered and filed into Dorothy's living room.

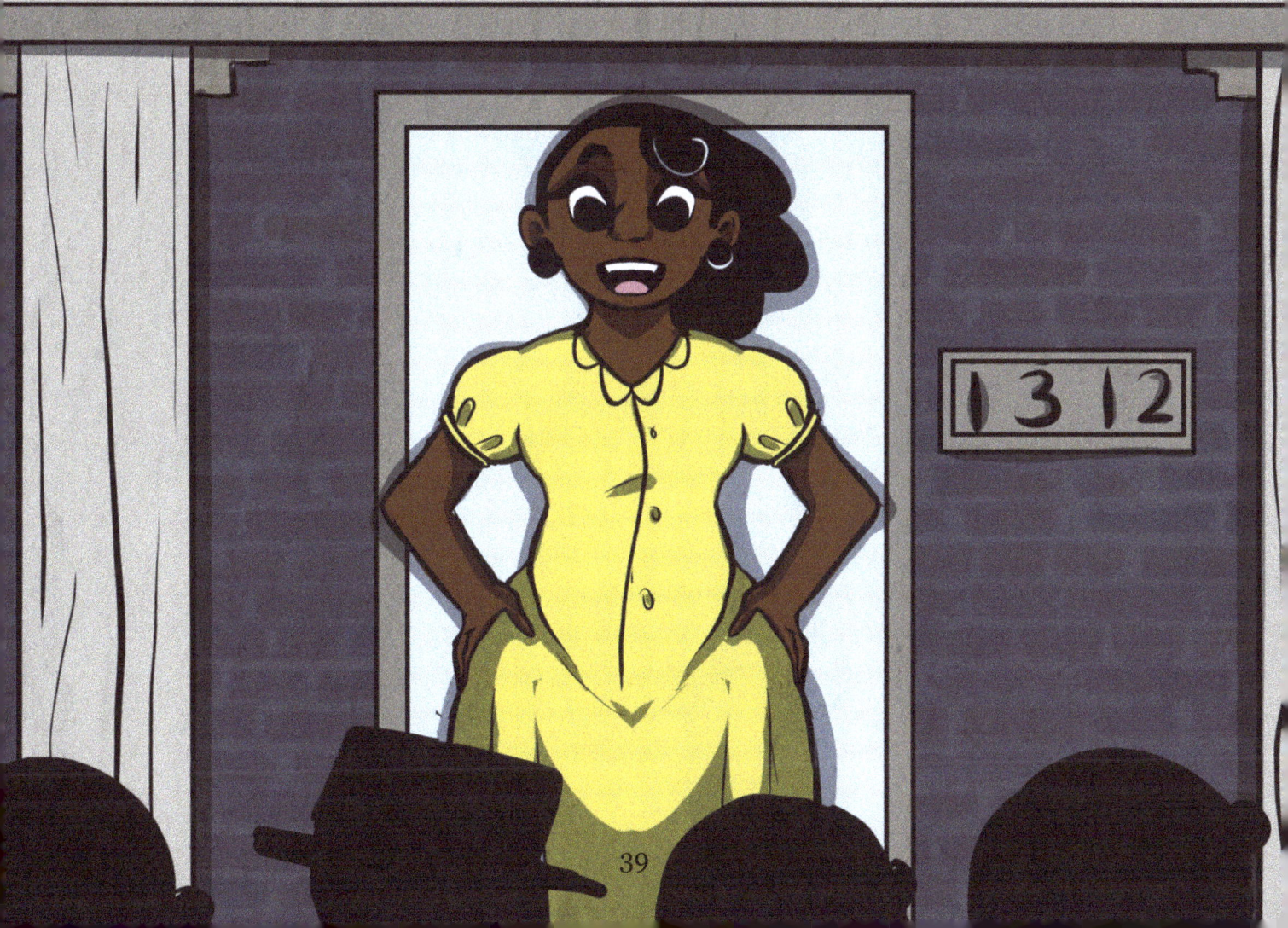

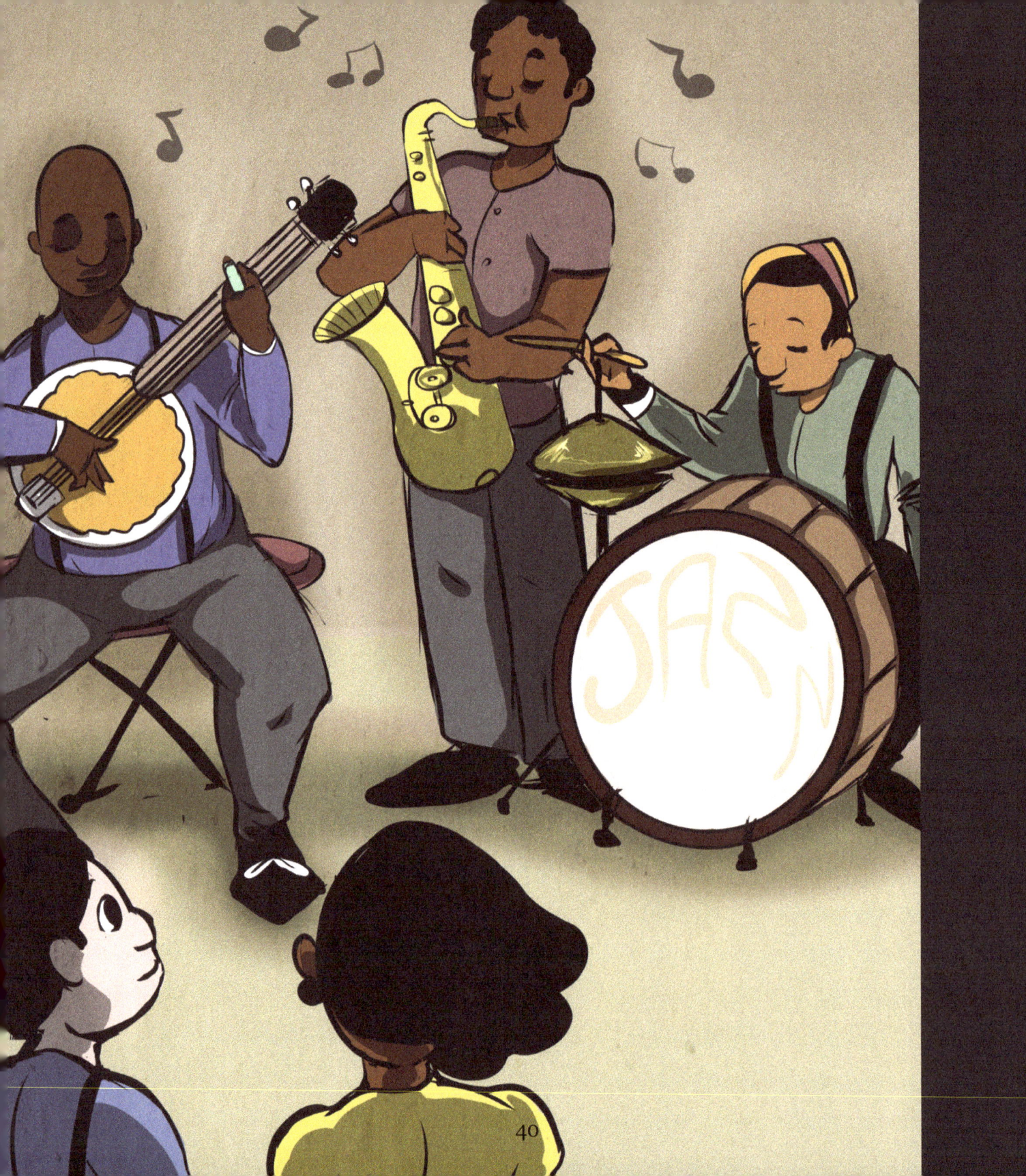

As George's eyes scanned the room for Dorothy, he felt someone grab his hand.

"What do you think of my Daddy's band?"

"They sound great. We should ask them to play at the next dance."

"You really want to come to another one after the night we had?"

"As long as *you're* there to dance with me."

Dorothy gave George a gentle nudge on the shoulder. "Thanks for gathering everyone up."

George nudged her back. "Thanks for saving the dance. And thanks for doing the lindy hop with me. Want to try again?"

"Yes, but this time I'm going to lead!" And with that Dorothy swung George onto the floor.

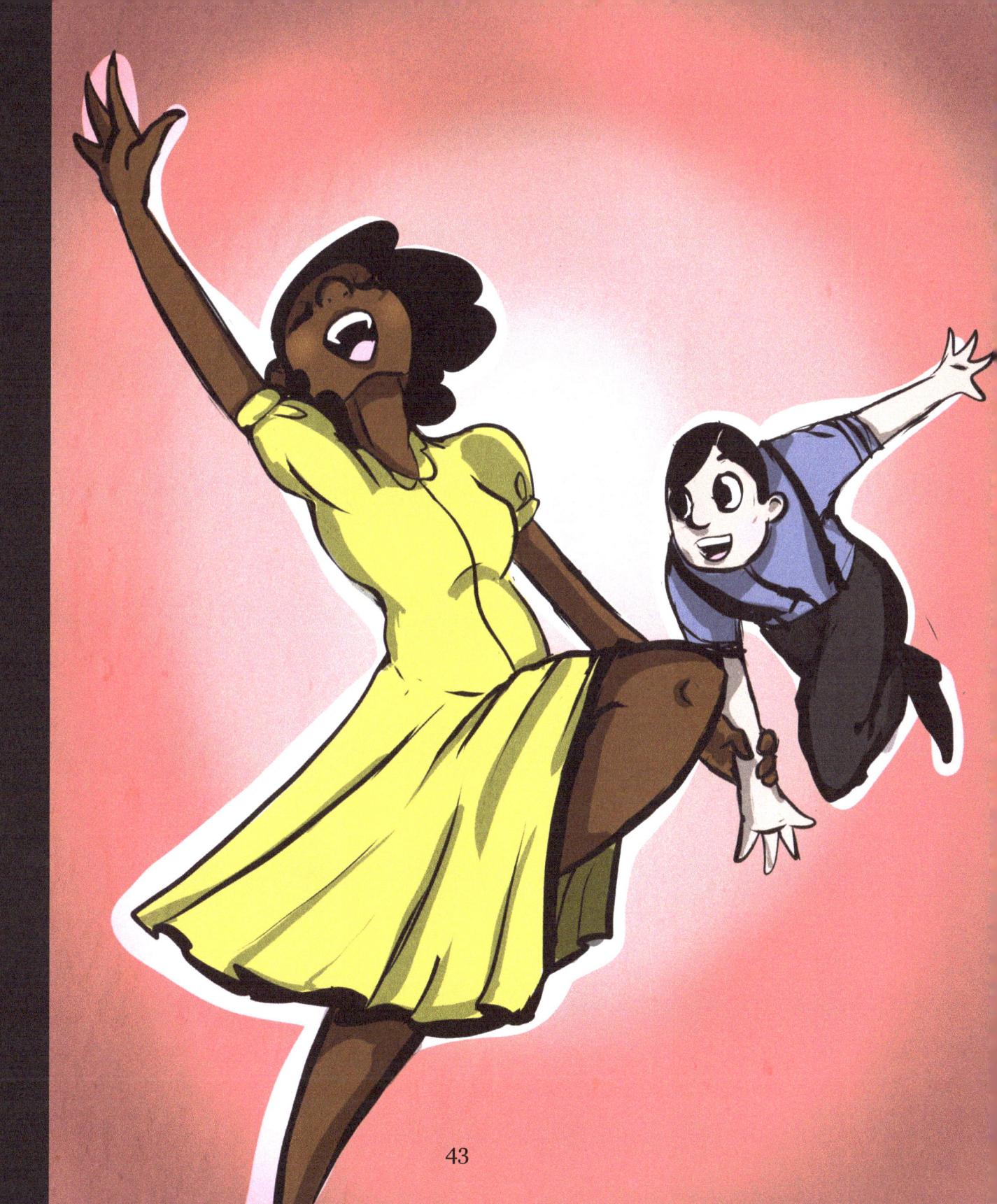

Historical Note

While this book is fiction, it's inspired by a real event. On the corner of James Street and Foreland Ave in the Northside of Pittsburgh, stands a building that's been part of the community since the late nineteenth century. It has functioned in a variety of different ways, starting off as *The International Social Lyceum* where labor organizers, socialists and many other neighborhood groups could hold meetings. It was also a dance hall, a restaurant, and most recently a jazz bar called the *James Street Gastropub and Speakeasy*.

According to Historian David Rosenburg, an undated notation was found in the building that stated, "police closed up a dance sponsored by the Young Workers League because of mixed people, colored and white" (Rosenberg, David. "Pittsburgh Lyceum home to labor, socialist groups." *Pennsylvania History Journal*, v. 27, Dec 2005.)

Segregation was the law of the land in the United States starting with Jim Crow Laws in the 1870's. Legal segregation wasn't completely abolished until the passing of the *Civil Rights Act of 1964*. This Act was passed because of the power of the Civil Rights movement, which came from ordinary people going to meetings, protests, and organizing their communities.

DISCUSSION QUESTIONS

1. What is your favorite type of music? Your favorite song? Your favorite dance move?

2. How did you feel when the police officers showed up to shut-down the dance?

3. In this story George struggles with deciding to help fight back against segregation and violence. Have you ever struggled when deciding to do something that you know is right? Have you ever been afraid to stand-up for yourself or your friends? What was that like?

4. Have you heard the phrase "white privilege"? What does that mean to you?

5. This story takes place in the 1930's when segregation was part of our laws. Even though segregation is not legal now, do you think something like this could still happen today? Why or why not?

6. Think about your own neighborhood. Is it mostly people who have the same color skin or the same ethnicity living around each other? What about your school? Your grocery store? Your playground?

7. What are some ways we can fight against segregation and discrimination that is happening today in our own communities?

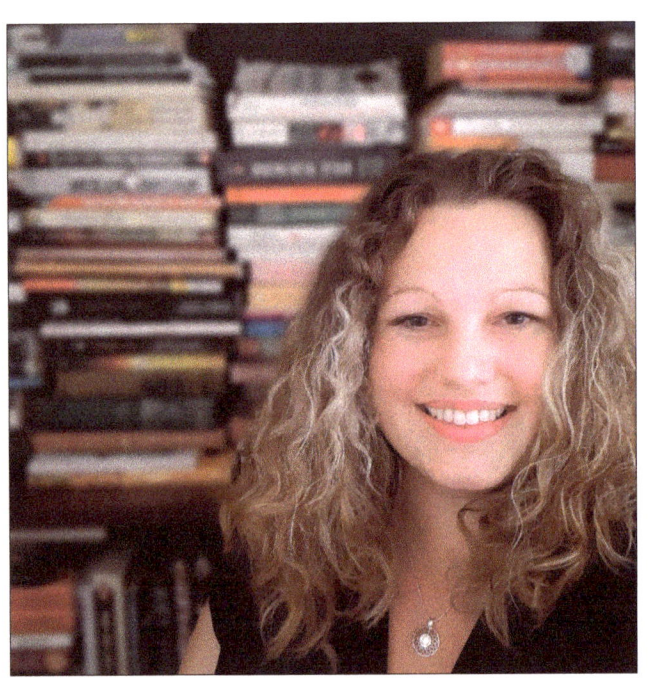

NICOLE MCCANDLESS *(Author)*

I was raised by a few hard-working, fiery women. They passed down a love of reading and gave me the confidence to put words on the page.

I've had many different jobs, including grocery store clerk, hostess, retail cashier, waitress, and labor organizer.

I recently dove into a life of writing and raising up two humans.

I love reading by myself in bed and with my kids on the floor. Other things I love include Ben, our sisters, being outside, dancing, singing, snacks, the changing of seasons, and sending people I love things in the mail.

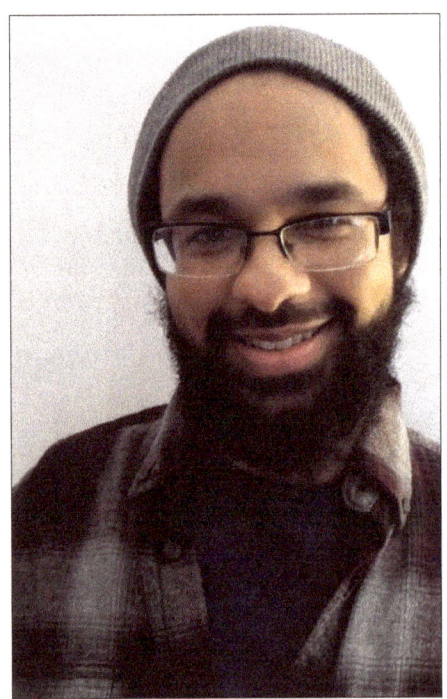

BYRON GRAMBY *(Illustrator)*

Art school dropout to graduating magna cum laude from Point Park with a Bachelors in Psychology. Not content to leave his stories in the trash, Byron has self-published four other children's stories over the years, along with two graphic novels.

When he's not creating children's books, he's taking a departure from children's books to write dark, ambient synth tracks or equally grim comics. You can find all of Byron's works on his website at " https://byrongramby.wordpress.com/

CHILDREN'S & YOUNG ADULT BOOKS

The Cabbage That Came Back
Stephen Pearl (Author)
Sara Pearl (Translator)
Rafael Pearl (Illustrator)

Down on James Street
Nicole McCandless (Author)
Byron Gramby (Illustrator)

For All/Para Todos
Alejandra Domenzain (Author)
Katherine Loh (Illustrator)
Irene Prieto de Coogan (Translator)

Freedom Soldiers
a YA novel, Katherine Williams

Good Guy Jake
Mark Torres (Author)
Yana Muraskho (Illustrator)
Madelin Arroyo (Translator)

Hats Off For Gabbie!
Marivir Montebon (Author)
Yana Murashko (Illustrator)
Laura Flores (Translator)

Jimmy's Carwash Adventure
Victor Narro (Author)
Yana Murashko (Illustrator)
Madelin Arroyo (Translator)

Joelito's Big Decision
Ann Berlak (Author)
Daniel Camacho (Illustrator)
Jose Antonio Galloso (Translator)

Manny & the Mango Tree
Ali Bustamante (Author)
Monica Lunot-Kuker (Illustrator)
Mauricio Niebla (Translator)

Margarito's Forest
Andy Carter (Author)
Allison Havens (Illustrator)
Omar Majeia (Translator)

Polar Bear Pete's Ice Is Melting!
(A 2021 release)
Timothy Sheard (Author)
Kayla Fils-Aime (Illustrator)
Madelin Arroyo (Translator)

Trailer Park,
JC Dillard (Author)
Anna Usacheva (Illustrator)
Madelin Arroyo (Translator)

CPSIA information can be obtained
at www.ICGtesting.com
Printed in the USA
BVHW020312070221
599335BV00003B/45